Health at a Glance: Europe 2010

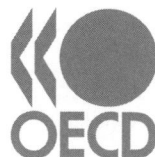

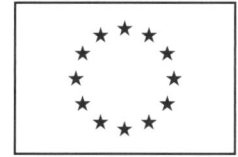

This work is published on the responsibility of the Secretary-General of the OECD. The opinions expressed and arguments employed herein do not necessarily reflect the official views of the OECD or of the governments of its member countries or those of the European Union.

Please cite this publication as:
OECD (2010), *Health at a Glance: Europe 2010*, OECD Publishing.
http://dx.doi.org/10.1787/health_glance-2010-en

ISBN 978-92-64-09030-9 (print)
ISBN 978-92-64-09031-6 (PDF)

Foreword

This first edition of Health at a Glance: Europe presents a set of key indicators on health and health systems across 31 countries – the 27 European Union member states, three European Free Trade Association countries (Iceland, Norway and Switzerland), and Turkey. The selection of indicators is based on the European Community Health Indicators (ECHI) shortlist – a set of indicators used by the European Commission to guide the development of health information systems in Europe. In addition, the publication provides detailed information on health expenditure trends across countries, building on the OECD's established expertise in this area.

This publication is a concrete example of the long and fruitful collaboration between the OECD and the European Commission in the development and reporting of health statistics. This collaboration also involves the World Health Organization (WHO).

The preparation of this report has been greatly facilitated by the increased co-operation in the collection of health statistics at the international level in recent years. A joint data collection between the OECD, Eurostat (the European statistical agency) and WHO was launched at the end of 2005 to improve the availability and comparability of data on health expenditure and financing, based on the System of Health Accounts. Building on the success of the joint Health Accounts collection, a new joint data collection between the three organisations was launched in 2010 to gather data on non-monetary health care statistics. These joint data collections are improving the comparability of data across countries, while reducing the data collection burden on national administrations.

Health at a Glance: Europe 2010 would not have been possible without the effort of national data correspondents from the 31 countries who have provided most of the data and the metadata presented in this report. The OECD and the European Commission would like to sincerely thank them for their contribution.

This publication was prepared by a team from the OECD Health Division under the co-ordination of Gaétan Lafortune and Michael de Looper. Chapter 1 and Chapter 2 were prepared by Michael de Looper and Valerie Moran, with a contribution from Carol Jagger and Jean-Marie Robine (Network on Health Expectancy, REVES) for the indicators related to life expectancy and healthy life years. Chapter 3 was prepared by Gaétan Lafortune and Gaëlle Balestat, with a contribution from Vladimir Stevanovic and Rie Fujisawa for the two indicators related to cancer care. Chapter 4 was written by David Morgan and Rebecca Bennetts. It is important to recognise the contribution of colleagues from Eurostat (in particular Elodie Cayotte and Albane Gourdol) and WHO-European Office (in particular Ivo Rakovac), who have shared some of the data presented in this publication. This publication benefited from comments from Mark Pearson (Head of OECD Health Division) and Nick Fahy, Fabienne Lefebvre and Federico Paoli (European Commission – DG Sanco).

Aart De Geus
Deputy Secretary-General
Organisation for Economic Co-operation
and Development

Paola Testori Coggi
Director-General
Directorate-General for Health and Consumers
European Commission

Table of Contents

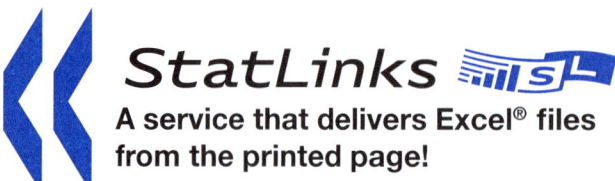

This book has...

StatLinks

A service that delivers Excel® files from the printed page!

Look for the *StatLinks* at the bottom right-hand corner of the tables or graphs in this book. To download the matching Excel® spreadsheet, just type the link into your Internet browser, starting with the *http://dx.doi.org* prefix.

If you're reading the PDF e-book edition, and your PC is connected to the Internet, simply click on the link. You'll find *StatLinks* appearing in more OECD books.

Acronyms

AIDS	Acquired immunodeficiency syndrome
ALOS	Average length of stay
AMI	Acute myocardial infraction
BMI	Body mass index
CAT (or CT)	Computed axial tomography (scanner)
EFTA	European Free Trade Association
EU	European Union
EU-SILC	European Union Statistics on Income and Living Conditions survey
GALI	Global activity limitation indicator
GDP	Gross domestic product
GP	General practitioner
HBSC	Health Behavior in School-aged Children survey
HIV	Human immunodeficiency virus
HLY	Healthy life years
IHD	Ischemic heart disease
ISIC	International Standard Industrial Classification
MRI	Medical resonance imaging
PPP	Purchasing power parities
SHA	System of Health Accounts
SIDS	Sudden infant death syndrome

Executive Summary

European countries have achieved major gains in population health over recent decades. Life expectancy at birth in European Union (EU) countries has increased by six years since 1980, while premature mortality has reduced dramatically. Improvements in living and working conditions and in some health-related behaviours have contributed greatly to these longevity gains, but progress in medical care also deserves much credit. Health systems are of growing size and complexity in European countries, and spending on health care has never been higher, consuming an ever-increasing share of national income.

This first edition of *Health at a Glance: Europe*, the result of a long-standing collaboration between the OECD and the European Commission, presents a set of key indicators of health and health systems in 31 European countries – the 27 member states of the European Union, and Iceland, Norway, Switzerland and Turkey. The selection of indicators has been based on the European Community Health Indicators (ECHI) shortlist, a list of indicators that has been developed by the European Commission to guide the development and reporting of health statistics (European Commission, 2010a). However, a number of indicators in this report differ from ECHI definitions because of data availability or constraints, or in some instances because ECHI indicators are not yet ready for implementation. The publication also provides detailed information on health expenditure and its financing, building on the OECD's established data collection and expertise in this area. The data presented in the publication come mainly from official national statistics, as gathered in *OECD Health Data*, the *Eurostat Statistics Database* and WHO-Europe's *Health for All Database*.

Health at a Glance: Europe 2010 presents evidence of wide variations across European countries in population health status, risk factors for health, the inputs, outputs and outcomes of health care systems, and levels of health expenditure and financing sources. It offers some explanation for these variations, providing a background to understand more fully the causes underlying such variations and to develop policy options to reduce gaps across countries. It should also be noted that while basic population breakdowns by sex and age are presented, this publication does not generally provide detail by sub-national regions, by socio-economic groups or by ethnic/racial groups. For many indicators, readers should keep in mind that there may be as much variation *within* a country as there is *across* countries.

Health status has improved dramatically
in European countries, although large gaps persist

- Life expectancy at birth in EU countries has increased by six years since 1980, reaching 78 years in 2007. On average across the 27 EU countries, life expectancy at birth for the three-year period 2005-07 stood at 74.3 years for men and 80.8 years for women. France had the highest life expectancy at birth for women (84.4 years), while Sweden had the highest life expectancy for men (78.8 years). Life expectancy at birth in the European Union was lowest in Romania for women (76.2 years) and Lithuania for men (65.1 years). The gap between countries with the highest and lowest life expectancies at birth is around eight years for women and 14 years for men.

- Whether the gains in life expectancy involve additional years of life lived in good health has important implications for health and long-term care systems in Europe. Healthy life years at birth is defined as the number of years of life in which a person's day-to-day activities are not limited by a condition or health problem. In 2005-07, healthy life years stood at 61.3 years for women and 60.1 years for men, on average, in the European Union. The gender gap is much smaller than for life expectancy, reflecting the fact that a higher proportion of women's lives are spent with activity limitations. Healthy life years at birth in 2005-07 was greatest in Malta for both men and women, and shortest in Latvia for women and Estonia for men.

- Life expectancy at age 65 has also increased substantially over the past decades in European countries. The average in 2005-07 for the 27 EU countries was 15.9 years for men and 19.5 years for women. As for life expectancy at birth, France had the highest life expectancy at age 65 for women (22.6 years) but also for men (18.1 years). Life expectancy at age 65 was lowest in Eastern Europe – in Latvia for men (12.7 years) and in Bulgaria for women (16.3 years).

- As is the case at birth, the gender gap for healthy life years at age 65 is much narrower than for life expectancy. In 2005-07, men were slightly favoured, at 8.4 years *versus* 8.1 years for women.

- It is difficult to estimate the relative contribution of the numerous medical and non-medical factors that might affect variations in (healthy) life expectancy. Higher national income is generally associated with higher life expectancy across European countries, although the relationship is less pronounced at higher levels of national income, suggesting a "diminishing return" after a certain level. Other determinants of health also play an important role.

Risk factors to health are changing

- Many EU countries have achieved remarkable progress in reducing tobacco consumption, although it is still a leading cause of early death. Much of this decline can be attributed to policies at national and EU level promoting public awareness campaigns, advertising bans and increased taxation. Less than 18% of adults in Sweden and Iceland now smoke daily, down from over 30% in 1980. However, almost 40% of adults in Greece continue to smoke on a daily basis. Smoking rates are also relatively high in Bulgaria, Ireland and the Netherlands.

- Alcohol consumption has also fallen in many European countries over the past three decades. Curbs on advertising, sales restrictions and taxation have proven to be effective measures to reduce alcohol consumption. Traditional wine-producing countries such as Italy, France and Spain have seen their alcohol consumption per capita drop substantially since 1980. On the other hand, consumption rose significantly in a number of countries including Ireland, the United Kingdom and some Nordic countries.

- More than half of the total adult population across the European Union are now overweight or obese. This is also true in 15 of the 27 EU countries. The prevalence of obesity – which presents greater health risks than overweight – varies from less than 10% in Romania, Switzerland and Italy to over 20% in the United Kingdom, Ireland, Malta and Iceland. On average across EU countries, 15.5% of the adult population is obese.

- The rate of obesity has more than doubled over the past 20 years in most EU countries for which data are available. The rapid increase occurred regardless of what the levels of obesity were two decades ago. Obesity more than doubled in both the Netherlands and the United Kingdom between 1988 and 2008, even though the rate in the Netherlands is currently less than half that of the United Kingdom.

- Because obesity is associated with higher risks of chronic illnesses, it is linked to significant additional health care costs. A recent study in England estimated that total costs linked to overweight and obesity could increase by as much as 70% between 2007 and 2015, and be 2.4 times higher by 2025 (Foresight, 2007).

Shortages of health workers is a concern in many countries

- There are concerns in many European countries about shortages of doctors. The number of doctors per capita varies greatly, and is lowest in Turkey, followed by Poland and Romania. Doctor numbers are also relatively low in the United Kingdom and Finland.

- Since 2000, the number of physicians per capita has however increased in all European countries, except the Slovak Republic. On average, the number grew from 3.0 doctors per 1 000 population in 2000 to 3.3 in 2008. It increased particularly rapidly in Ireland, rising by nearly 50%. A large part of this increase was due to the recruitment of foreign-trained physicians, with the share of foreign-trained doctors tripling during that period. Similarly, the number of doctors per capita in the United Kingdom increased by 30% between 2000 and 2008, rising from 2.0 per 1 000 population to 2.6.

- In contrast, there has been virtually no growth in the number of doctors per capita in France and Italy since 2000. Following a reduction in the number of new entrants in medical schools during the 1980s and 1990s, the number of doctors per capita in Italy peaked in 2002, and has declined since then. In France, the number peaked in 2005, and the decline is expected to continue over the next ten years.

- In nearly all countries, the balance between general practitioners and specialists has changed over past decades, with the number of specialists increasing much more rapidly. As a result, there are more specialists than generalists in most countries, except Romania and Portugal. This may be explained by a reduced attractiveness in the traditional mode of practice of general/family practitioner, as well as a growing remuneration gap. The slow growth or reduction in the number of generalists per capita raises concerns about access to primary care. Many countries are considering ways to improve the attractiveness of general practice as well as developing new roles for other health care providers, such as nurses.

● There are also concerns about shortages of nurses in many European countries. Nurses play an important role in providing health care not only in traditional settings such as hospitals and long-term care institutions but increasingly in primary care, especially in offering care to the chronically ill, and in patients' homes. In 2008, there were about 15 nurses per 1 000 population in Finland, Iceland, Ireland and Switzerland, and slightly fewer in Denmark and Norway. Turkey had the fewest nurses, followed by Greece, Bulgaria and Cyprus, at less than five per 1 000 population.

● Since 2000, the number of nurses per capita has increased in all European countries, except Lithuania and the Slovak Republic. The increase was particularly large in Portugal, Spain, France and Switzerland.

Growing health expenditure puts pressure on government budgets

● Health expenditure has risen in all European countries, often increasing at a faster rate than economic growth, resulting in a rising share of GDP allocated to health. In 2008, EU countries spent, on average, 8.3% of their GDP on health, up from 7.3% in 1998. However, the share of GDP allocated to health spending varies considerably across countries, ranging from less than 6% in Cyprus and Romania to more than 10% in France, Switzerland, Germany and Austria.

● In some countries, the recent economic downturn resulted in a marked increase in the ratio of health spending to GDP. In Ireland, the percentage of GDP devoted to health increased from 7.5% in 2007 to 8.7% in 2008. In Spain, it rose from 8.4% to 9.0%.

● In 2008, Norway spent the most on health per capita among European countries, with spending of about EUR 4 300. Switzerland, Luxembourg and Austria were the next highest spending countries. Most northern and western European countries spend between EUR PPP 2 500 and 3 500 per person, that is, 10% to 60% more than the EU average. Those countries spending below the EU average are eastern and southern European countries such as Turkey, Romania, Bulgaria, Poland and Hungary.

● Health expenditure per capita tends to be positively correlated with GDP per capita, although the association is stronger among European countries with low GDP per capita. Even for countries with similar levels of GDP per capita, there can be substantial differences in health expenditure. For example, Spain and France have similar GDP per capita, but Spain spends less than 80% of the level of France on health.

● Health systems are sometimes criticised for being overly focused on "sick care": for treating the ill, but not doing enough to prevent illness. Only around 3% of current health expenditure is spent on prevention and public health programmes on average in EU countries.

● The public sector is the main source of health financing in all European countries, except Cyprus. On average, nearly three-quarter of all health spending was publicly financed in 2008, through general taxation or social security contributions. In Luxembourg, the Czech Republic, the Nordic countries (except Finland), the United Kingdom and Romania, public financing accounted for more than 80% of all health expenditure.

- The size and composition of private financing differs across countries. In most countries, it is in the form of out-of-pocket payments by patients. Private health insurance accounts for only around 3-4% of total health expenditure on average across EU countries. However, in some countries, it plays a significant role. In Germany, it provides primary coverage for certain population groups. In France, private health insurance finances 13% of overall spending, but provides complementary and supplementary coverage in a universal public system.

- Given the current need to reduce budget deficits in many countries, governments may be faced with difficult policy choices in the short-term. They may either have to curb the growth of public spending on health, cut spending in other areas, or raise taxes or social security contributions to reduce their deficits. Improving productivity within the health sector may help to reconcile these pressures, for example through more rigorous assessment of health technologies or increased used of information and communication technologies ("eHealth"). These initiatives may also have the added benefit of improving the quality of care, which is another area of collaboration between the OECD and the European Commission.

Résumé

Les pays européens ont accompli d'importants progrès en matière de santé au cours des dernières décennies. Dans les pays de l'Union européenne, l'espérance de vie à la naissance a augmenté de six ans depuis 1980, tandis que la mortalité précoce a fortement reculé. Si l'amélioration des conditions de vie et de travail, ainsi que de certains comportements vis-à-vis de la santé, a joué un rôle majeur dans l'augmentation de la longévité, les progrès de la médecine doivent également être salués. Les systèmes de santé dans les pays européens occupent une place de plus en plus importante et les dépenses consacrées aux soins de santé n'ont jamais été aussi élevées, représentant une part croissante du revenu national.

Cette première édition de *Panorama de la santé : Europe*, fruit d'une collaboration de longue date entre l'OCDE et la Commission européenne, propose un ensemble d'indicateurs clés de la santé et des systèmes de santé dans 31 pays européens, à savoir les 27 États membres de l'Union européenne, l'Islande, la Norvège, la Suisse et la Turquie. La sélection d'indicateurs s'appuie sur la liste des indicateurs de santé de la Communauté européenne (*European Community Health Indicators* – ECHI), élaborée par la Commission européenne pour étayer la production et la publication de statistiques sur la santé (Commission européenne, 2010a). Certains des indicateurs diffèrent parfois des définitions retenues pour la liste ECHI pour des questions de disponibilité des données. Dans d'autres cas, les indicateurs ECHI ne sont pas encore prêts à être mis en œuvre. Par ailleurs, la publication fournit également des informations détaillées sur les dépenses de santé et leur financement, en s'appuyant sur l'expérience de l'OCDE en matière de collecte de données dans ce domaine. Les informations présentées dans *Panorama de la santé : Europe* sont essentiellement issues de sources statistiques nationales officielles, notamment d'*Éco-Santé OCDE*, de la base de données statistique Eurostat et de la base de données *Santé pour tous* de l'OMS-Europe.

Panorama de la santé : Europe 2010 montre qu'il existe d'importants écarts entre les pays européens en termes d'état de santé de la population, de facteurs de risques pour la santé, d'intrants, d'extrants et de résultats des systèmes de santé, et de niveaux des dépenses de santé et des sources de financement. L'étude propose des explications à ces écarts, en fournissant le contexte nécessaire pour mieux comprendre leurs causes sous-jacentes. Il convient aussi de noter que si des disparités par sexe et par âge sont présentées, cette publication ne fournit généralement pas d'informations sur les disparités par région, par groupe socioéconomique ou par groupe ethnique. Pour de nombreux indicateurs, le lecteur doit garder à l'esprit que les variations peuvent être aussi importantes *au sein* d'un même pays qu'*entre* les pays.

L'état de santé s'est amélioré de manière
remarquable dans les pays européens,
même si des écarts importants persistent

- Dans les pays de l'UE, l'espérance de vie à la naissance s'est allongée de six ans depuis 1980, pour atteindre 78 ans en 2007. En moyenne dans les 27 pays de l'UE, l'espérance de vie à la naissance pour la période 2005-07 s'élevait à 74.3 ans pour les hommes et à 80.8 ans pour les femmes. La France affiche l'espérance de vie à la naissance la plus longue pour les femmes (84.4 ans), tandis que l'espérance de vie la plus longue pour les hommes est observée en Suède (78.8 ans). Au sein de l'Union européenne, c'est en Roumanie que l'espérance de vie à la naissance est la plus courte pour les femmes (76.2 ans) et en Lituanie pour les hommes (65.1 ans). L'écart entre les pays à l'espérance de vie la plus longue et ceux où l'espérance de vie est la plus courte s'établit à 8 ans environ pour les femmes et à 14 ans pour les hommes.

- Il importe de savoir si l'allongement de l'espérance de vie implique des années de vie supplémentaires en bonne santé, parce que cela a des répercussions majeures sur les systèmes de santé et de soins de longue durée en Europe. L'espérance de vie en bonne santé à la naissance est définie ici comme le nombre d'années de vie au cours desquelles les activités quotidiennes de l'individu ne sont pas limitées par une maladie ou un problème de santé. En 2005-07, l'espérance de vie en bonne santé s'établissait à 61.3 ans pour les femmes et 60.1 ans pour les hommes en moyenne dans l'Union européenne. L'écart hommes-femmes est donc bien moindre qu'en ce qui concerne l'espérance de vie, ce qui tient au fait qu'une plus forte proportion de la vie des femmes est marquée par des limitations de leur activité. En 2005-07, c'est à Malte que l'espérance de vie en bonne santé était la plus longue à la fois pour les hommes et pour les femmes, tandis que la Lettonie affichait l'espérance de vie en bonne santé la plus courte pour les femmes et l'Estonie pour les hommes.

- L'espérance de vie à l'âge de 65 ans s'est aussi considérablement accrue en Europe au cours des dernières décennies. En 2005-07, elle s'élevait en moyenne dans les 27 pays de l'UE à 15.9 ans pour les hommes et 19.5 ans pour les femmes. Comme pour l'espérance de vie à la naissance, la France se distingue par l'espérance de vie à 65 ans la plus longue pour les femmes (22.6 ans) mais aussi pour les hommes (18.1 ans). Au contraire, c'est en Europe de l'Est que l'espérance de vie à 65 ans est la plus courte : en Lettonie pour les hommes (12.7 ans) et en Bulgarie pour les femmes (16.3 ans).

- Comme pour l'espérance de vie à la naissance, l'écart hommes-femmes s'agissant de l'espérance de vie en bonne santé à 65 ans est bien plus restreint que pour l'espérance de vie : en 2005-07, les hommes étaient légèrement avantagés, avec 8.4 ans contre 8.1 ans pour les femmes.

- Il est difficile d'estimer la contribution relative des multiples facteurs médicaux et non médicaux susceptibles d'influencer les écarts dans l'espérance de vie (en bonne santé). Un revenu national élevé est généralement associé à une meilleure espérance de vie dans les pays européens, quoique cette corrélation soit moins prononcée pour les niveaux de revenu élevés, ce qui suggère un « rendement décroissant » à partir d'un certain seuil. D'autres déterminants de la santé jouent également un rôle clé.

Les facteurs de risques évoluent

- De nombreux pays de l'UE ont accompli des progrès remarquables dans la lutte contre le tabagisme, même s'il demeure l'une des principales causes de mortalité précoce. Cette réussite peut en grande partie être attribuée aux mesures mises en œuvre à l'échelle nationale et européenne pour promouvoir les campagnes de sensibilisation publique, les interdictions de publicité et la hausse des taxes. En Suède et en Islande, moins de 18 % des adultes fument désormais quotidiennement, contre plus de 30 % en 1980. En revanche, près de 40 % des adultes continuent de fumer quotidiennement en Grèce. Le taux de tabagisme demeure également élevé en Bulgarie, en Irlande et aux Pays-Bas.

- La consommation d'alcool a également diminué dans nombre de pays européens ces 30 dernières années. Les restrictions sur la publicité et les ventes et la hausse des taxes se sont avérées des outils efficaces pour réduire la consommation d'alcool. Les pays traditionnellement producteurs de vin, comme l'Italie, la France et l'Espagne, ont vu la consommation d'alcool par habitant chuter fortement depuis 1980. À l'inverse, la consommation a sensiblement augmenté dans plusieurs pays comme l'Irlande, le Royaume-Uni et certains pays nordiques.

- Plus de la moitié de la population adulte totale de l'Union européenne est désormais en situation de surpoids ou d'obésité. C'est également le cas dans 15 des 27 pays de l'UE. La prévalence de l'obésité – qui présente des risques pour la santé supérieurs à ceux du surpoids – est comprise entre moins de 10 % en Roumanie, en Suisse et en Italie à plus de 20 % au Royaume-Uni, en Irlande, à Malte et en Islande. En moyenne dans les pays de l'UE, 15.5 % de la population adulte est obèse.

- Le taux d'obésité a plus que doublé ces 20 dernières années dans la plupart des pays de l'UE pour lesquels des données sont disponibles. Cette progression rapide est intervenue indépendamment des taux d'obésité observés il y a 20 ans. L'obésité a plus que doublé aux Pays-Bas et au Royaume-Uni entre 1988 et 2008, même si le taux observé aux Pays-Bas est actuellement inférieur de plus de moitié à celui du Royaume-Uni.

- L'obésité étant associée à une augmentation des risques de maladie chronique, elle entraîne un coût supplémentaire important au niveau des soins de santé. Selon une étude récente réalisée en Angleterre, la hausse du coût représenté par le surpoids et l'obésité pourrait aller jusqu'à 70 % entre 2007 et 2015 et il pourrait être 2.4 fois plus élevé d'ici à 2025 (Foresight, 2007).

La pénurie de professionnels de santé est un sujet d'inquiétude dans de nombreux pays

- De nombreux pays européens s'inquiètent d'une pénurie de médecins. Le nombre de médecins par habitant varie fortement entre les pays ; il atteint son niveau le plus bas en Turquie, suivie par la Pologne et la Roumanie. Il est également relativement bas au Royaume-Uni et en Finlande.

- Depuis 2000, le nombre de médecins par habitant a néanmoins augmenté dans tous les pays européens, à l'exception de la Slovaquie. En moyenne, il est passé de 3.0 médecins pour 1 000 habitants en 2000 à 3.3 en 2008. Cette progression a été particulièrement rapide en Irlande, avec une hausse de près de 50 %. Ceci s'explique en grande partie par le recrutement de médecins formés à l'étrangers : le nombre de médecins formés à l'étranger a en effet triplé sur la période. De la même façon, le nombre de médecins par habitant au Royaume-Uni a progressé de 30 % entre 2000 et 2008, passant de 2.0 pour 1 000 habitants à 2.6.

- À l'inverse, le nombre de médecins par habitant est resté pratiquement inchangé en France et en Italie depuis 2000. Après une baisse du nombre de nouveaux inscrits en école de médecine dans les années 80 et 90, le nombre de médecins par habitant a atteint son point le plus haut en 2002 en Italie, pour s'orienter ensuite à la baisse. En France, il a touché son plus haut niveau en 2005 et la baisse devrait se poursuivre au cours des dix prochaines années.

- Dans la quasi-totalité des pays, le rapport entre médecins généralistes et spécialistes a évolué au cours des dernières décennies, le nombre de spécialistes ayant progressé bien plus rapidement. Par conséquent, les spécialistes sont aujourd'hui plus nombreux que les généralistes dans la plupart des pays, à l'exception de la Roumanie et du Portugal. Ce phénomène peut s'expliquer par une diminution de l'attrait offert par le mode traditionnel de la pratique du médecin généraliste/de famille, ainsi que par un écart de rémunération croissant. La hausse limitée, voire la baisse, du nombre de généralistes par habitant suscite des inquiétudes quant à l'accès aux soins primaires. De nombreux pays étudient des moyens pour renforcer l'attractivité de la médecine générale et pour concevoir de nouveaux rôles pour d'autres professionnels de santé, comme le personnel infirmier.

- Par ailleurs, de nombreux pays européens sont touchés par une pénurie de personnel infirmier. Les infirmiers jouent un rôle important dans la prestation des soins de santé non seulement dans le cadre traditionnel de l'hôpital ou des établissements de soins de longue durée mais aussi, de plus en plus, dans les soins primaires, notamment auprès des malades chroniques et dans les traitements à domicile. En 2008, on comptait environ 15 infirmières pour 1 000 habitants en Finlande, en Islande, en Irlande et en Suisse, et un peu moins au Danemark et en Norvège. La Turquie est le pays où l'on compte le moins d'infirmiers, suivie par la Grèce, la Bulgarie et Chypre, avec moins de 5 pour 1 000 habitants.

- Depuis 2000, le nombre de personnel infirmier par habitant a progressé dans tous les pays européens, à l'exception de la Lituanie et de la Slovaquie. Cette progression est particulièrement importante au Portugal, en Espagne, en France et en Suisse.

L'augmentation des dépenses de santé pèse sur les budgets nationaux

- Les dépenses de santé ont augmenté dans tous les pays européens, la plupart du temps à un rythme supérieur à celui de la croissance économique, ce qui se traduit par une augmentation de la part du PIB allouée à la santé. En 2008, les pays de l'UE ont consacré en moyenne 8.3 % de leur PIB aux dépenses de santé, contre 7.3 % en 1998. Néanmoins, la part du PIB allouée aux dépenses de santé varie considérablement entre les pays, de moins de 6 % à Chypre et en Roumanie à plus de 10 % en France, en Suisse, en Allemagne et en Autriche.

- Dans certains pays, la récession récente a provoqué une hausse notable de la part des dépenses de santé dans le PIB. Ainsi, en Irlande, la part du PIB consacrée à la santé a progressé de 7.5 % en 2007 à 8.7 % en 2008. En Espagne, elle est passée de 8.4 % à 9.0 %.

- En 2008, la Norvège est le pays qui affiche les dépenses de santé par habitant les plus élevées parmi les pays européens, à 4 300 EUR environ, suivie par la Suisse, le Luxembourg et l'Autriche. La plupart des pays d'Europe du Nord et de l'Ouest ont dépensé entre 2 500 et 3 500 EUR par habitant, ce qui est supérieur de 10 à 60 % à la moyenne de l'UE. Les pays où les dépenses de santé sont inférieures à la moyenne de l'UE sont les pays d'Europe de l'Est et du Sud comme la Turquie, la Roumanie, la Bulgarie, la Pologne et la Hongrie.

- Les dépenses de santé par habitant présentent généralement une corrélation positive avec le PIB par habitant, même si celle-ci est plus étroite dans les pays européens caractérisés par un PIB par habitant relativement bas. Cependant, même dans les pays au PIB par habitant équivalent, on peut observer des écarts importants en matière de dépenses de santé. Par exemple, l'Espagne et la France affichent un PIB par habitant assez proche, mais les dépenses de santé de l'Espagne représentent moins de 80 % de celles de la France.

- On déplore parfois que les systèmes de santé soient trop tournés sur les soins aux malades, c'est-à-dire qu'ils sont davantage axés sur le traitement des maladies plutôt que sur leur prévention. En moyenne dans les pays de l'UE, seulement 3 % environ des dépenses de santé sont consacrées à la prévention et aux programmes de santé publique.

- Le secteur public représente la principale source de financement de la santé dans tous les pays européens, à l'exception de Chypre. En moyenne, près de 75 % des dépenses de santé totales étaient financées par les fonds publics en 2008, au moyen des recettes fiscales ou des cotisations de sécurité sociale. Au Luxembourg, en République tchèque, dans les pays nordiques (hors Finlande), au Royaume-Uni et en Roumanie, le financement public couvre les dépenses de santé à hauteur de plus de 80 %.

- L'ampleur et la composition du financement privé varient selon les pays. Généralement, il prend la forme d'une participation financière par les patients. L'assurance maladie privée ne représente que 3-4 % seulement des dépenses de santé totales en moyenne dans les pays de l'UE. Toutefois, dans certains pays, elle a un rôle de financement important. Ainsi, elle assure une couverture primaire à certaines catégories de population en Allemagne. En France, l'assurance maladie privée finance 13 % des dépenses totales mais elle fournit une couverture complémentaire et supplémentaire dans le cadre d'un régime public universel.

- De nombreux pays étant actuellement soucieux de réduire leurs déficits budgétaires, les pouvoirs publics seront confrontés à des choix difficiles à court terme. Ils pourraient en effet être contraints soit de freiner la croissance des dépenses publiques de santé, soit de réduire les dépenses dans d'autres secteurs, ou soit d'augmenter les impôts ou les cotisations de sécurité sociale, pour réduire leurs déficits. Des gains de productivité et d'efficience dans le secteur de la santé pourraient contribuer à alléger les pressions, par exemple au moyen d'une évaluation plus rigoureuse des technologies de santé ou d'un recours accru aux technologies de l'information et de la communication. Ces initiatives pourraient en outre permettre d'améliorer la qualité des soins, ce qui constitue un autre axe important de collaboration entre l'OCDE et la Commission européenne.

Health at a Glance: Europe 2010
© OECD 2010

Introduction

H*ealth at a Glance: Europe 2010* presents key indicators of health and health systems in 31 European countries, including the 27 European Union member states, three EFTA countries (Iceland, Norway and Switzerland), and Turkey. It builds on the format used in the OECD's previous editions of *Health at a Glance* to provide comparable information on important public health issues in Europe. The indicators have been selected on the basis of the European Community Health Indicators (ECHI) shortlist (European Commission, 2010a; ECHIM, 2010). However, in some instances, this report deviates from the formal ECHI definitions because of issues related to data availability and comparability. Detailed information is also provided in this publication on health expenditure and financing trends, based on the OECD's long-standing data collection in this area. All indicators are presented in the form of easy-to-read figures and explanatory text.

Structure of the publication

The structure of *Health at a Glance: Europe 2010* generally reflects the structure of the European Community Health Indicators. It is divided into four chapters:

- Chapter 1 on *Health Status* highlights the variations across countries in life expectancy and healthy life expectancy, and also presents other indicators of causes of mortality and morbidity, including both communicable and non-communicable diseases.

- Chapter 2 on *Determinants of Health* focuses on non-medical determinants of health related to modifiable lifestyles and behaviours among children and adults, such as smoking and alcohol drinking, nutrition habits, physical activity, and overweight and obesity.

- Chapter 3 on *Health Care Resources, Services and Outcomes* reviews some of the inputs, outputs and outcomes of health care systems, including the supply of doctors and nurses, different types of equipment used for diagnosis or treatment, and the provision of a range of services to prevent the transmission of communicable diseases or to treat acute conditions. It concludes with a review of care related to cancer, focusing on the coverage of screening programmes and survival rates for two types of cancer: breast and cervical cancer.

- Chapter 4 on *Health Expenditure and Financing* examines trends in health spending across European countries, both overall and for different types of health services and goods, including pharmaceuticals. It also looks at how these health services and goods are paid for and the different mix between public funding, private health insurance, and direct out-of-pocket payments by households.

An annex provides some additional tables on the demographic and economic context within which different health systems operate.

Presentation of indicators

Each of the topics covered in this publication is presented over two pages. The first provides a brief commentary highlighting the key findings conveyed by the data, defines the indicator(s) and discloses any significant national variations from that definition which might affect data comparability. On the facing page is a set of figures. These typically show current levels of the indicator and, where possible, trends over time. In some cases, an additional figure relating the indicator to another variable is included. The average in the figures includes only European Union (EU) countries, and is calculated as the unweighted average of those EU countries presented (up to 27, if there is full data coverage).

Data limitations

Limitations in data comparability are indicated both in the text (in the box related to "Definition and deviations") as well as in footnotes to charts.

Readers interested in using the data presented in this publication for further analysis and research are encouraged to consult the full documentation of definitions, sources and methods contained in *OECD Health Data 2010* for all OECD member countries. This information is available at *www.oecd.org/health/healthdata*.

For the six non-OECD member countries (Bulgaria, Cyprus, Latvia, Lithuania, Malta and Romania), readers should consult the *Eurostat Database* at *http://epp.eurostat.ec.europa.eu/portal/page/portal/statistics/search_database*.

Readers interested in an interactive presentation of the ECHI indicators can also consult the SANCO health indicators tool at *www.ec.europa.eu/health/indicators/indicators/index_en.htm*.

Population figures

The population figures presented in the annex and used to calculate rates per capita in this publication come from the *OECD Labour Force Statistics Database* (as of May 2010) for OECD member countries, and refer to mid-year estimates. For the six non-OECD member countries, the data come from the *Eurostat Demographics Database* (as of July 2010), and refer to estimates at the beginning of the year. Population estimates are subject to revision, so they may differ from the latest population figures released by national statistical offices.

Note that some countries such as France and the United Kingdom have overseas colonies, protectorates and territories. These populations are generally excluded. The calculation of GDP per capita and other economic measures may, however, be based on a different population in these countries, depending on the data coverage.

Country codes (ISO codes)

Austria	AUT	Lithuania	LTU
Belgium	BEL	Luxembourg	LUX
Bulgaria	BGR	Malta	MLT
Cyprus[1]	CYP	Netherlands	NLD
Czech Republic	CZE	Norway	NOR
Denmark	DNK	Poland	POL
Estonia	EST	Portugal	PRT
Finland	FIN	Romania	ROM
France	FRA	Slovak Republic	SVK
Germany	DEU	Slovenia	SVN
Greece	GRC	Spain	ESP
Hungary	HUN	Sweden	SWE
Iceland	ISL	Switzerland	CHE
Ireland	IRL	Turkey	TUR
Italy	ITA	United Kingdom	GBR
Latvia	LVA		

1. *Note by Turkey:* The information in this document with reference to "Cyprus" relates to the Southern part of the Island. There is no single authority representing both Turkish and Greek Cypriot people on the Island. Turkey recognises the Turkish Republic of Northern Cyprus (TRNC). Until a lasting and equitable solution is found within the context of United Nations, Turkey shall preserve its position concerning the "Cyprus" issue.

   Note by all the European Union member states of the OECD and the European Commission: The Republic of Cyprus is recognised by all members of the United Nations with the exception of Turkey. The information in this document relates to the area under the effective control of the Government of the Republic of Cyprus.

Chapter 1

Health Status

Life expectancy at birth continues to increase remarkably in EU countries, reflecting reductions in mortality rates at all ages. These gains in longevity can be attributed to a number of factors, including rising living standards, improved lifestyle and better education, as well as greater access to quality health services. Other factors, such as better nutrition, sanitation and housing also play a role, particularly in countries with developing economies (OECD, 2004).

Average life expectancy at birth for the years 2005-07 across the 27 countries of the European Union reached 74.3 years for men and 80.8 years for women (Figure 1.1.1), a rise of approximately three years for men and two years for women over the decade from 1995-97. In around 70% of EU countries, life expectancy at birth in 2005-07 exceeded 80 years for women and 77 years for men. France had the highest life expectancy at birth for women (84.4 years), while Sweden had the highest life expectancy at birth for men (78.8 years). At the other end of the scale, life expectancy at birth in the European Union was lowest in Romania for women (76.2 years) and Lithuania for men (65.1 years). The gap between EU countries with the highest and lowest life expectancies at birth is around eight years for women and 14 years for men.

The gender gap in life expectancy at birth in 2005-07 stood at 6.5 years, almost one year less than a decade earlier. However, this average hides a huge range among countries with the smallest gender gap in life expectancy at birth in the United Kingdom and Cyprus (4.1 years) and the largest in Lithuania (12.1 years). The recent narrowing of the gender gap in life expectancy can be attributed at least partly to the narrowing of differences in risk-increasing behaviours between men and women, such as smoking, accompanied by sharp reductions in mortality rates from cardio-vascular diseases among men.

On average for EU countries healthy life years (HLY) at birth in 2005-07 was 61.3 years for women and 60.1 years for men. HLY at birth in 2005-07 was greatest in Malta for both men and women, and shortest in Latvia for women and Estonia for men (Figure 1.1.1). The spread of values for HLY at birth among EU countries were much greater than for life expectancy, being 17.0 years for women and 19.5 years for men, but there was a much smaller absolute difference between men and women (2.5 years). Since the HLY indicator has only recently been developed, there is as yet no long time series.

In contrast to the 6.5 year gap in life expectancy at birth for EU countries on average, the gender gap in HLY at birth was 1.2 years in 2005-07. For life expectancy at birth the gender gap is always in favour of women. However, eight countries had a gender gap in HLY at birth which favoured men, the greatest being 1.9 years more HLY for men at birth than women in the Netherlands. Of the remaining countries, Poland had the largest gender gap in HLY at birth favouring women.

Higher national income (as measured by GDP per capita) is generally associated with higher life expectancy at birth, although the relationship between GDP and HLY is less obvious (Figure 1.1.2). There is a modest positive relationship, with increasing GDP per capita associated with increasing HLY, although it is less pronounced at higher levels of national income. There are also notable differences in HLY between EU countries with similar income per capita. Sweden and the United Kingdom have higher, and Finland and Estonia lower HLY than would be predicted by their GDP alone. Similarly, Figure 1.1.3 shows the relationship between HLY at birth and health spending per capita. Higher health spending per capita is generally associated with higher HLY.

Definition and deviations

Life expectancy measures how long, on average, people would live based on a given set of age-specific death rates. However, the actual age-specific death rates of any particular birth cohort cannot be known in advance. If age-specific death rates are falling (as has been the case over the past decades in EU countries), actual life spans will be higher than life expectancy calculated with current death rates.

Healthy life years (HLY) at a particular age are the number of years spent free of activity limitation. They are calculated by Eurostat for each EU country using the Sullivan method (Sullivan, 1971). The underlying health measure is the Global Activity Limitation Indicator (GALI) which comes from the European Union Statistics on Income and Living Conditions (EU-SILC) survey. The GALI measures limitation in usual activities. The questionnaire responses used in Denmark differ slightly, resulting in an under-estimation of activity limitation. Data are not available for Bulgaria, Switzerland and Turkey.

Comparing trends in HLY and life expectancy can show whether extra years of life are healthy years. However, valid comparisons depend on the underlying health measure being truly comparable. While HLY is the most comparable indicator to date, there are still problems with translation of the GALI question, although it does appear to satisfactorily reflect other health and disability measures (Jagger et al., 2010).

1.1.1. Life expectancy and healthy life years (HLY) at birth, by gender, 2005-07

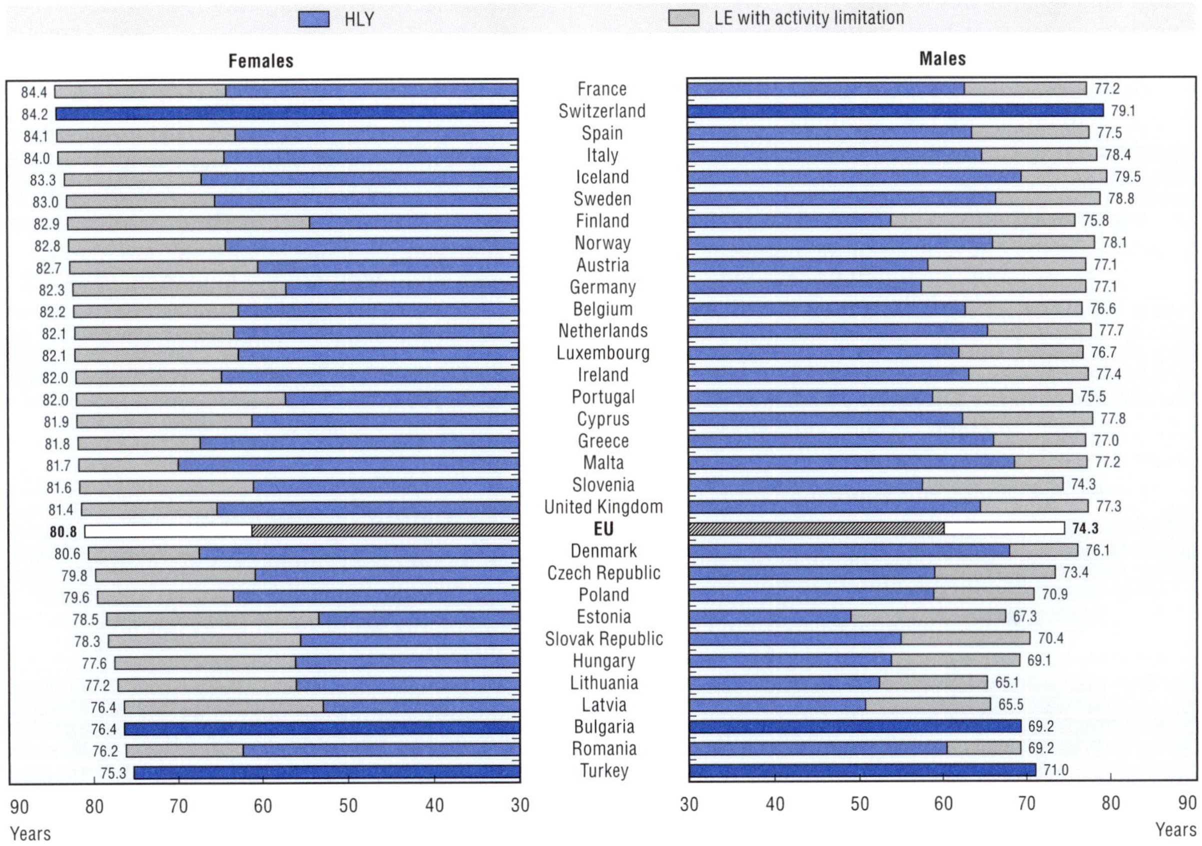

HLY
LE with activity limitation
Females
Males
France 84.4 77.2
Switzerland 84.2 79.1
Spain 84.1 77.5
Italy 84.0 78.4
Iceland 83.3 79.5
Sweden 83.0 78.8
Finland 82.9 75.8
Norway 82.8 78.1
Austria 82.7 77.1
Germany 82.3 77.1
Belgium 82.2 76.6
Netherlands 82.1 77.7
Luxembourg 82.1 76.7
Ireland 82.0 77.4
Portugal 82.0 75.5
Cyprus 81.9 77.8
Greece 81.8 77.0
Malta 81.7 77.2
Slovenia 81.6 74.3
United Kingdom 81.4 77.3
EU 80.8 74.3
Denmark 80.6 76.1
Czech Republic 79.8 73.4
Poland 79.6 70.9
Estonia 78.5 67.3
Slovak Republic 78.3 70.4
Hungary 77.6 69.1
Lithuania 77.2 65.1
Latvia 76.4 65.5
Bulgaria 76.4 69.2
Romania 76.2 69.2
Turkey 75.3 71.0
90 80 70 60 50 40 30
30 40 50 60 70 80 90
Years

Source: European Health and Life Expectancy Information System (EHLEIS); *OECD Health Data 2010*; *Eurostat Statistics Database*.

StatLink http://dx.doi.org/10.1787/888932335400

1.1.2. Healthy life years (HLY) at birth, 2005-07 and GDP per capita, 2007

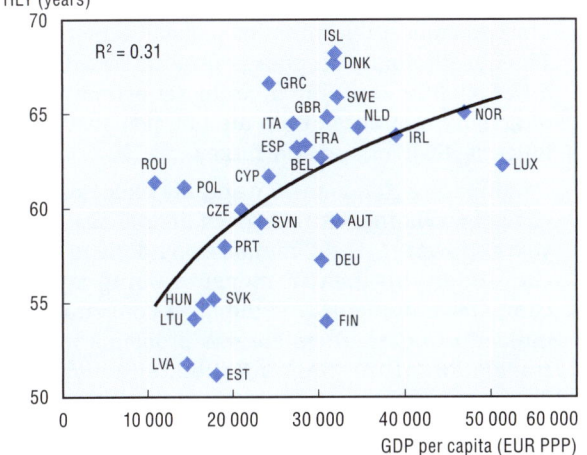

HLY (years)
R^2 = 0.31
ISL
DNK
GRC
SWE
GBR
NLD
NOR
ITA
IRL
ESP
FRA
ROU
BEL
LUX
POL
CYP
CZE
SVN
AUT
PRT
DEU
HUN
SVK
LTU
FIN
LVA
EST
70
65
60
55
50
0
10 000
20 000
30 000
40 000
50 000
60 000
GDP per capita (EUR PPP)

Source: European Health and Life Expectancy Information System (EHLEIS); *OECD Health Data 2010*; *Eurostat Statistics Database*; WHO.

StatLink http://dx.doi.org/10.1787/888932335419

1.1.3. Healthy life years (HLY) at birth, 2005-07 and health spending per capita, 2007

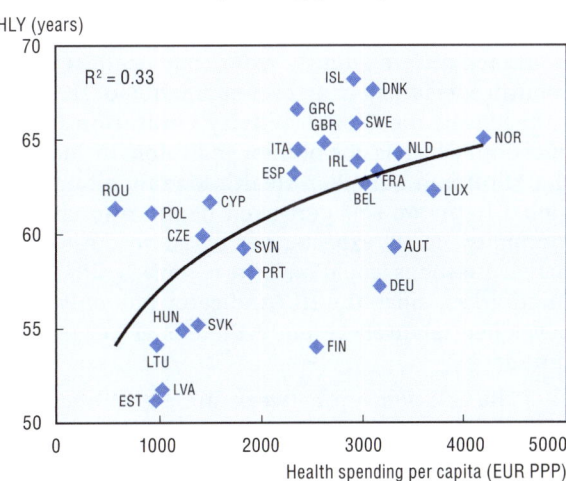

HLY (years)
R^2 = 0.33
ISL
DNK
GRC
GBR
SWE
ITA
NLD
NOR
IRL
ESP
FRA
ROU
BEL
LUX
POL
CYP
CZE
SVN
AUT
PRT
DEU
HUN
SVK
LTU
FIN
LVA
EST
70
65
60
55
50
0
1000
2000
3000
4000
5000
Health spending per capita (EUR PPP)

Source: European Health and Life Expectancy Information System (EHLEIS); *OECD Health Data 2010*; *Eurostat Statistics Database*; WHO.

StatLink http://dx.doi.org/10.1787/888932335438

Life expectancy at age 65 has increased significantly among both women and men over the past several decades in all EU countries. Some of the factors explaining the gains in life expectancy at age 65 include advances in medical care combined with greater access to health care, healthier lifestyles and improved living conditions before and after people reach age 65.

The average life expectancy at age 65 years in 2005-07 for the 27 countries of the European Union was 15.9 years for men and 19.5 years for women (Figure 1.2.1). As for life expectancy at birth, France had the highest life expectancy at age 65 for women (22.6 years) but also for men (18.1 years). Life expectancy at age 65 in the European Union was lowest in Eastern Europe – in Latvia for men (12.7 years) and in Bulgaria for women (16.3 years).

The average gender gap in life expectancy at age 65 in 2005-07 stood at 3.6 years, down from the previous decade by 0.4 years. Greece had the smallest gender gap of two years and Estonia the largest at 5.1 years.

Gains in longevity at older ages in recent decades in EU countries, combined with the trend reduction in fertility rates are contributing to a steady rise in the proportion of older persons in EU countries (see Annex Tables A.2 and A.4). Whether longer life expectancy is accompanied by good health and functional status among ageing populations has important implications for health and long-term care systems.

As is the case for HLY at birth, HLY at age 65 in 2005-07 for EU countries was similar for men and women, being 8.4 years for men and 8.1 years for women. HLY at age 65 in 2005-07 was greatest in Denmark and shortest in Estonia for both men and women (Figure 1.2.1). It should be noted though, that the question used to measure activity limitation in Denmark differs slightly from that used in other countries, resulting in an over-estimation of HLY. HLY is based on the Global Activity Limitation (GALI) question, which is one of three indicators included in the Minimum European Health Module along with global items on self-perceived health and chronic morbidity. Health expectancies based on these alternative questions would rank the countries differently. In addition, since the HLY indicator has only been developed relatively recently, there is as yet no long time series.

The relationship between life expectancy and HLY at age 65 is not clear-cut (Figure 1.2.2). Higher life expectancy at age 65 is generally associated with higher HLY, but the relationship is less pronounced for women than for men. Longer life expectancy at age 65 does not necessarily imply more HLY.

Contrary to life expectancy where the rankings for men and women are different, there is a close association between HLY at age 65 for men and women. At the overall EU level, this consistency between the number of years spent free of activity limitation (HLY) between men and women at birth and at age 65 is true also for intermediate ages. Women's longer life expectancy at all ages are more often years spent with activity limitation. Lower HLY at age 50 across EU countries has been shown to be associated with lower GDP and with higher long-term unemployment and lower life-long learning for men (Jagger et al., 2008).

Definition and deviations

Life expectancy measures how long, on average, people would live based on a given set of age-specific death rates. However, the actual age-specific death rates of any particular birth cohort cannot be known in advance. If age-specific death rates are falling (as has been the case over the past decades in EU countries), actual life spans will be higher than life expectancy calculated with current death rates.

Healthy life years (HLY) at a particular age are the number of years spent free of activity limitation. They are calculated by Eurostat for each EU country using the Sullivan method (Sullivan, 1971). The underlying health measure is the Global Activity Limitation Indicator (GALI) which comes from the European Union Statistics on Income and Living Conditions (EU-SILC) survey. The GALI measures limitation in usual activities. The questionnaire responses used in Denmark differ slightly, resulting in an under-estimation of activity limitation. Data are not available for Bulgaria, Switzerland and Turkey.

Comparing trends in HLY and life expectancy can show whether extra years of life are healthy years. However, valid comparisons depend on the underlying health measure being truly comparable. While HLY is the most comparable indicator to date, there are still problems with translation of the GALI question, although it does appear to satisfactorily reflect other health and disability measures (Jagger et al., 2010).

1.2.1. Life expectancy and healthy life years (HLY) at 65, by gender, 2005-07

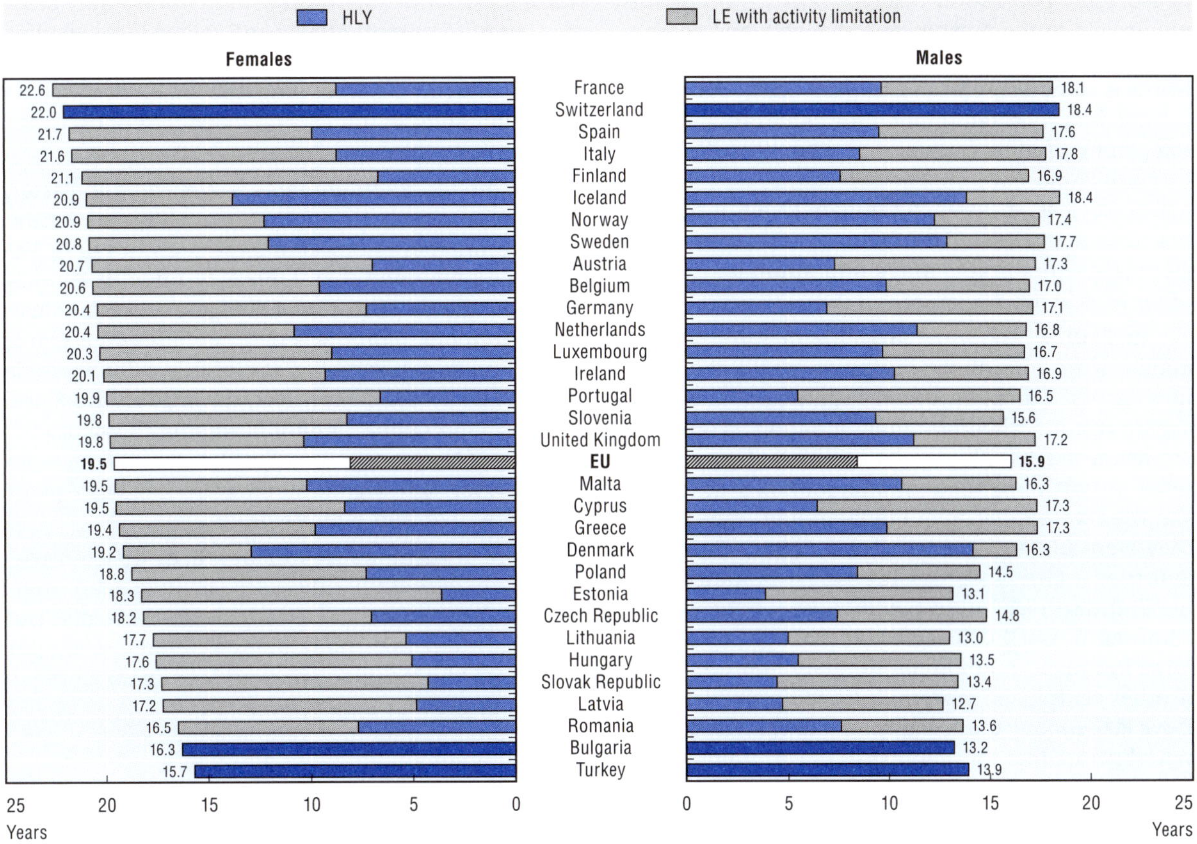

■ HLY   ▢ LE with activity limitation

Females

Value	Country	Value
22.6	France	18.1
22.0	Switzerland	18.4
21.7	Spain	17.6
21.6	Italy	17.8
21.1	Finland	16.9
20.9	Iceland	18.4
20.9	Norway	17.4
20.8	Sweden	17.7
20.7	Austria	17.3
20.6	Belgium	17.0
20.4	Germany	17.1
20.4	Netherlands	16.8
20.3	Luxembourg	16.7
20.1	Ireland	16.9
19.9	Portugal	16.5
19.8	Slovenia	15.6
19.8	United Kingdom	17.2
19.5	**EU**	**15.9**
19.5	Malta	16.3
19.5	Cyprus	17.3
19.4	Greece	17.3
19.2	Denmark	16.3
18.8	Poland	14.5
18.3	Estonia	13.1
18.2	Czech Republic	14.8
17.7	Lithuania	13.0
17.6	Hungary	13.5
17.3	Slovak Republic	13.4
17.2	Latvia	12.7
16.5	Romania	13.6
16.3	Bulgaria	13.2
15.7	Turkey	13.9

Males

Years (25 20 15 10 5 0 — 0 5 10 15 20 25) Years

Source: European Health and Life Expectancy Information System (EHLEIS); *Eurostat Statistics Database*; OECD Health Data 2010.

StatLink ⬛ http://dx.doi.org/10.1787/888932335457

1.2.2. Relationship between life expectancy and healthy life years (HLY) at 65, 2005-07

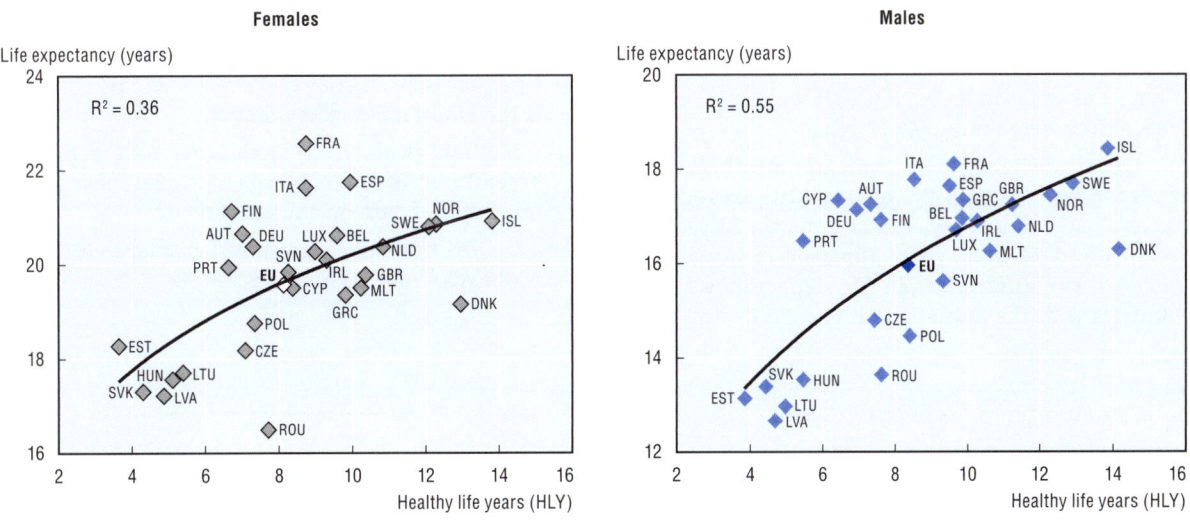

Females

Males

Source: European Health and Life Expectancy Information System (EHLEIS); *Eurostat Statistics Database*; OECD Health Data 2010.

StatLink ⬛ http://dx.doi.org/10.1787/888932335476

Mortality rates are one of the most common measures of population health. Statistics on deaths remain one of the most widely available and comparable sources of information on health. Registering deaths is compulsory in all European Union countries, and the data collected through the process of registration can be used by statistical and health authorities to monitor diseases and health status, and to plan health services. In order to compare levels of mortality across countries and over time, the data need to be aggregated in suitable ways and standardised for differences in age-structure.

In 2008 there were large variations in age-standardised total mortality rates for all causes of death across European Union countries. Death rates were lowest in Switzerland, Italy, Iceland and Spain, at 520 deaths per 100 000 population or less (Figure 1.3.1). Rates in northern, western and southern European countries were lower than the EU average rate of 696. They were highest in central and eastern European countries – Lithuania and Latvia, for instance, had age-standardised rates twice those of the lowest countries at over 1 000 deaths per 100 000 population. Rates in Bulgaria, Romania, Hungary and a number of other central and eastern European countries were above 800. Among these countries, only Slovenia had a mortality rate that was lower than the EU average.

Male mortality rates were lowest in Iceland, Switzerland and Sweden, and high in Lithuania, Latvia and Estonia. Female rates were low in France, Spain and Switzerland, and high in Bulgaria, Romania and Lithuania. A significant gender gap exists in mortality rates (Figure 1.3.1). Across all EU countries, the male mortality rate was, on average, 70% higher than the female rate in 2008. But large differences exist among countries – in Estonia, Lithuania and Latvia, male rates were more than twice those of females, whereas in Iceland, the United Kingdom and Greece they were around 40% higher.

Lower mortality rates translate into higher life expectancies. In 2005-07, average life expectancy across all EU countries was approximately 81 years for females and 74 years for males (see Indicator 1.1). However, the differences in life expectancy among countries with the lowest and highest mortality rates

are in the order of eight years for females and 12 years for males. Some important causes of mortality below the age of 65 years that may be avoided through effective evidence-based public health measures include ischemic heart disease, lung cancer, alcohol-related mortality, suicide, transport accidents, cervical cancer and AIDS (Cayotte and Buchow, 2009).

Although mortality rates in Central and Eastern Europe are still comparatively high, significant declines have occurred in a number of these countries since 1994 (Figures 1.3.2 and 1.3.3). Mortality rates in Estonia, Slovenia, the Czech Republic, Hungary and Poland have fallen by more than 30%, a decline that is greater than the EU average. Ireland has also seen a fall in mortality rates of over 50%. In contrast, declines in the Slovak Republic and Lithuania have been small. Declines in a number of Nordic countries (Sweden, Iceland) have also been modest, although these countries began the period with rates that were already low.

The leading causes of death in EU countries include cardiovascular diseases (such as heart attack and stroke), and cancer. Deaths from these diseases, plus selected external causes of death (transport accidents and suicide), are examined more closely in the following four indicators.

1.3.1. Mortality rates from all causes of death, 2008 (or nearest year available)

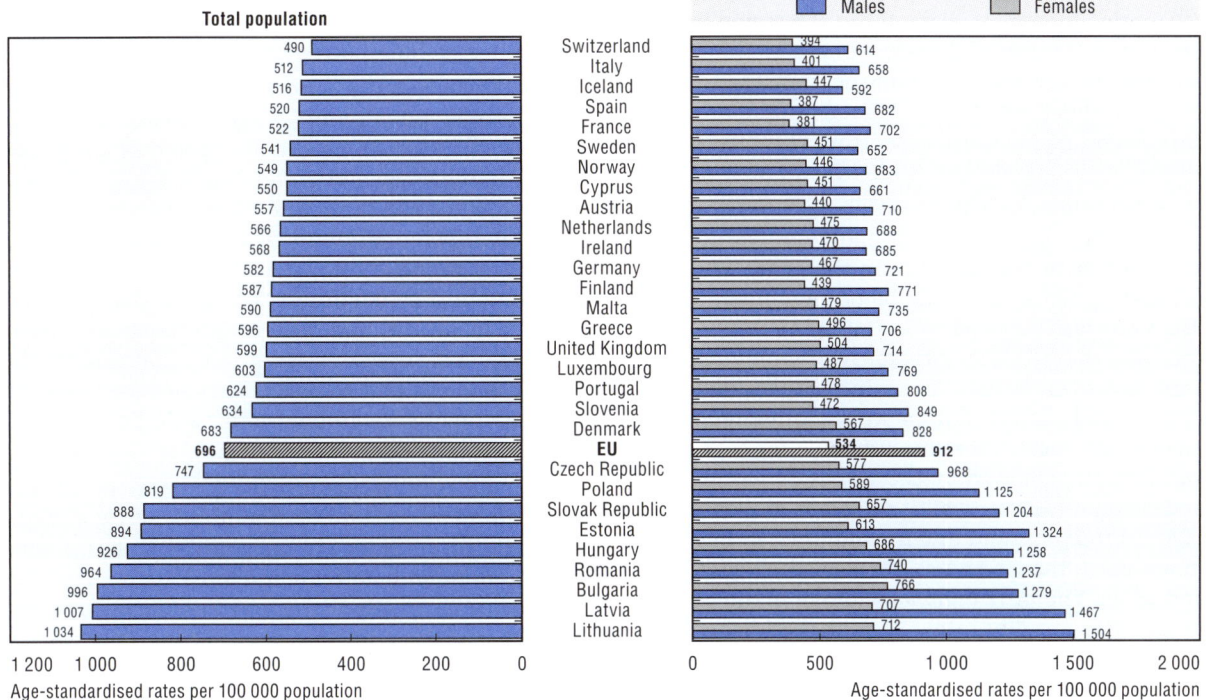

Source: Eurostat Statistics Database. Data are age-standardised to the WHO European standard population.

StatLink ᴍꜱ🔗 http://dx.doi.org/10.1787/888932335495

1.3.2. Decline in all cause mortality rates, 1994-2008 (or nearest year available)

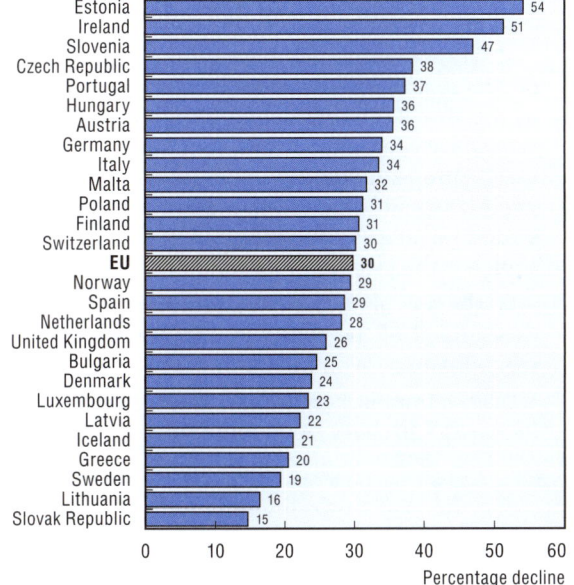

Source: Eurostat Statistics Database. Data are age-standardised to the WHO European standard population.

StatLink ᴍꜱ🔗 http://dx.doi.org/10.1787/888932335514

1.3.3. Trends in all cause mortality rates, selected EU countries, 1994-2008

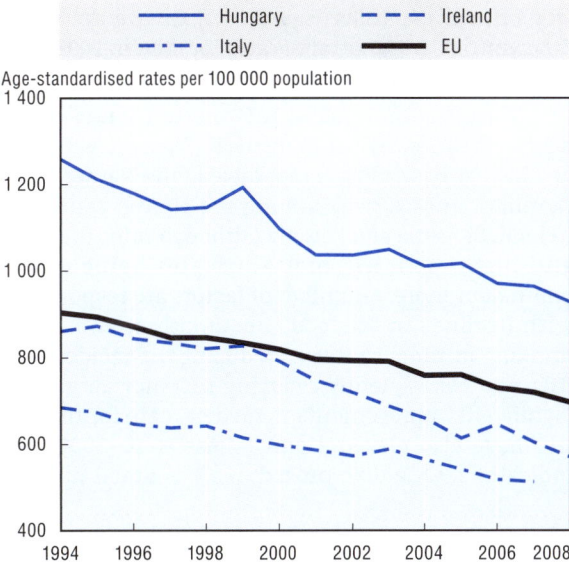

Source: Eurostat Statistics Database. Data are age-standardised to the WHO European standard population.

StatLink ᴍꜱ🔗 http://dx.doi.org/10.1787/888932335533

Cardiovascular diseases are the main cause of mortality in almost all European Union countries, accounting for 40% of all deaths in the region in 2008. They cover a range of diseases related to the circulatory system, including ischemic heart disease (known as IHD, or heart attack) and cerebro-vascular disease (or stroke). Together, IHD and stroke comprise 60% of all cardiovascular deaths, and caused one-quarter of all deaths in EU countries in 2008.

Ischemic heart disease is caused by the accumulation of fatty deposits lining the inner wall of a coronary artery, restricting blood flow to the heart. IHD alone was responsible for 15% of all deaths in EU countries in 2008. Mortality from IHD varies considerably, however, across EU countries (Figure 1.4.1). Central and eastern European countries report the highest IHD mortality rates, Lithuania for both males and females, followed by Latvia, the Slovak Republic and Estonia. IHD mortality rates are also relatively high in Finland, Malta and Ireland, with rates several times higher than in France, Portugal, the Netherlands and Spain. There are regional patterns to the variability in IHD mortality rates. Besides the Netherlands, the countries with the lowest IHD mortality rates are four countries located in Southern Europe: France, Portugal, Spain and Italy, with Greece also having low rates. This lends support to the commonly held hypothesis that there are underlying risk factors, such as diet, which explain differences in IHD mortality across countries.

Death rates are much higher for men than for women in all countries (Figure 1.4.1). On average across EU countries, IHD mortality rates for men in 2008 were nearly two times greater than for women.

Since the mid-1990s, IHD mortality rates have declined in nearly all countries (Figure 1.4.3). The decline has been most remarkable in the Netherlands, Denmark and Norway among the Nordic countries, Ireland, Slovenia and Estonia (although rates there are still high), with IHD mortality rates being cut by one-half or more. A number of factors are responsible, with declines in tobacco consumption, and heavy drinking in some countries reducing the incidence of IHD, and consequently reducing IHD mortality rates. Significant improvements in medical care for treating IHD have also played a part (Moïse et al., 2003) (see Indicator 3.9 "Cardiac procedures"). A small number of countries, however, have seen little or no decline since 1994. In the Slovak Republic, mortality rates have increased slightly. Declines in Poland, Hungary and Lithuania have been moderate, at under 20%.

Stroke is another important cause of mortality in EU countries, accounting for about 10% of all deaths in 2008. It is caused by the disruption of the blood supply to the brain, and in addition to being an important cause of mortality, the disability burden from stroke is substantial (Moon et al., 2003). As with IHD, there are large variations in stroke mortality rates across countries (Figure 1.4.2). Again, the rates are highest in central and eastern European countries, including Bulgaria, Romania, Latvia, Lithuania, the Slovak Republic and Hungary. They are the lowest in Switzerland, France, Iceland and the Netherlands.

Looking at trends over time, stroke mortality has decreased in all EU countries (except the Slovak Republic and Poland) since 1994, with a more pronounced fall after 1999 (Figure 1.4.4). Rates have declined by one-half or more in Italy, Estonia, Portugal, Austria, Germany and the Czech Republic. As with IHD, the reduction in stroke mortality can be attributed at least partly to a reduction in risk factors. Tobacco smoking and hypertension are the main modifiable risk factors for stroke. Improvements in medical treatment for stroke have also increased survival rates.

Definition and deviations

Mortality rates are based on numbers of deaths registered in a country in a year divided by the size of the corresponding population. The rates have been directly age-standardised to the WHO European standard population to remove variations arising from differences in age structures across countries and over time. The source is the Eurostat Statistics Database.

Mathers et al. (2005) have provided a general assessment of the coverage, completeness and reliability of data on causes of death.

Deaths from ischemic heart disease are classified to ICD-10 codes I20-I25, and stroke to I60-I69.

1.4.1. Ischemic heart disease, mortality rates, 2008 (or nearest year available)

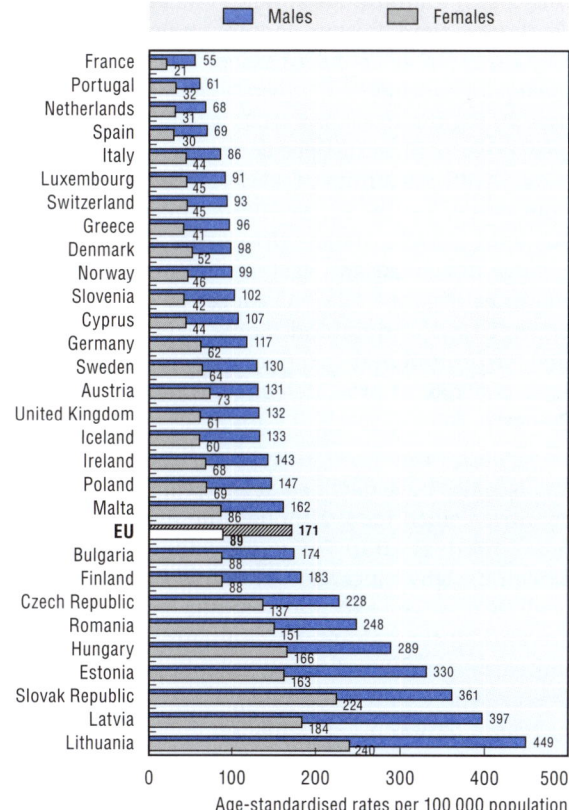

Source: Eurostat Statistics Database. Data are age-standardised to the WHO European standard population.

StatLink ⟨⟨⟨⟩⟩⟩ http://dx.doi.org/10.1787/888932335552

1.4.2. Stroke, mortality rates, 2008 (or nearest year available)

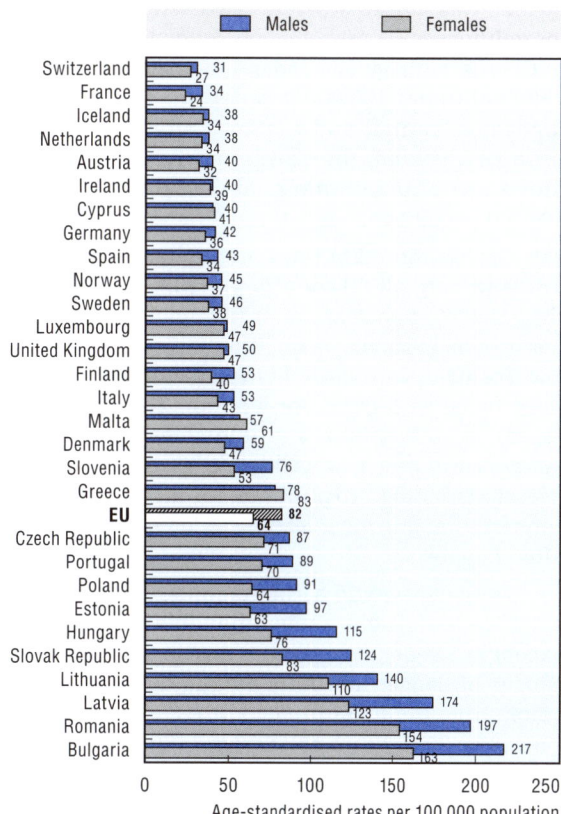

Source: Eurostat Statistics Database. Data are age-standardised to the WHO European standard population.

StatLink ⟨⟨⟨⟩⟩⟩ http://dx.doi.org/10.1787/888932335571

1.4.3. Trends in ischemic heart disease mortality rates, selected EU countries, 1994-2008

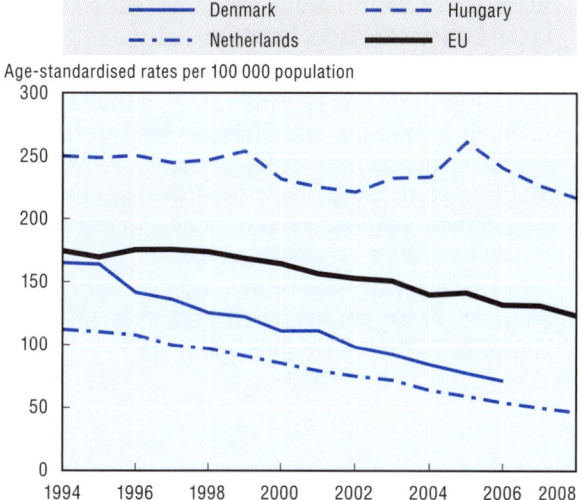

Source: Eurostat Statistics Database. Data are age-standardised to the WHO European standard population.

StatLink ⟨⟨⟨⟩⟩⟩ http://dx.doi.org/10.1787/888932335590

1.4.4. Trends in stroke mortality rates, selected EU countries, 1994-2008

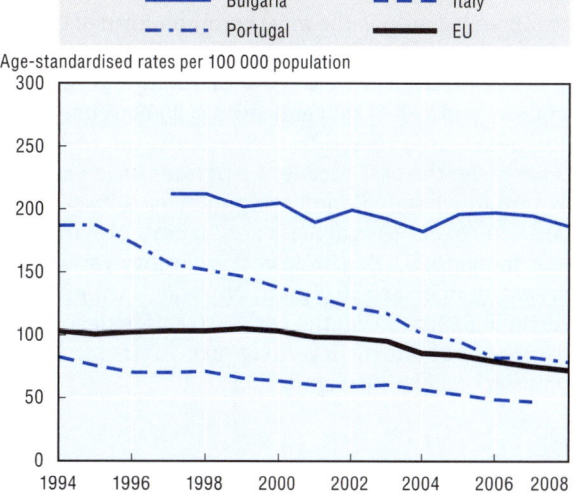

Source: Eurostat Statistics Database. Data are age-standardised to the WHO European standard population.

StatLink ⟨⟨⟨⟩⟩⟩ http://dx.doi.org/10.1787/888932335609

Cancer is the second leading cause of mortality in EU countries (after diseases of the circulatory system), accounting for 26% of all deaths in 2008. Cancer mortality rates for the total population were the lowest in Cyprus, Finland, Switzerland and Sweden, at under 150 deaths per 100 000 population. They were the highest in central and eastern European countries (Hungary, Poland, the Czech and Slovak Republics, Slovenia) and Denmark, above 200 deaths per 100 000 population.

Cancer mortality rates are higher for men than for women in all EU countries (Figure 1.5.1). In 2008, the gender gap in death rates from cancer was particularly wide in Latvia, Spain, Estonia, France, Lithuania and Portugal, with mortality rates among men more than twice as high as for women. This gap can be explained partly by the greater prevalence of risk factors among men, as well as the lesser availability or use of screening programmes for different types of cancers affecting men, leading to lower survival rates after diagnosis.

Lung cancer still accounts for the greatest number of cancer deaths among men in all EU countries, except in Sweden. Lung cancer is also one of the main causes of cancer mortality among women. Tobacco smoking is the most important risk factor for lung cancer. In 2008, death rates from lung cancer among men were the highest in central and eastern European countries (Hungary, Poland, Estonia, Latvia, Lithuania and others) (Figure 1.5.2). These are all countries where smoking rates among men are relatively high. Death rates from lung cancer among men are low in Nordic countries (Sweden, Iceland, Finland and Norway) as well as in Cyprus, countries with low smoking rates among men (see Indicator 2.6). Denmark and Iceland, however, have high rates of lung cancer mortality among women.

Breast cancer is the most common form of cancer among women in all EU countries (Ferlay et al., 2010). It accounted for 31% of cancer incidence among women, and 17% of cancer deaths in 2008. While there has been an increase in incidence rates of breast cancer over the past decade, death rates have declined or remained stable, indicating increases in survival rates due to earlier diagnosis and/or better treatments (see Indicator 3.13). The lowest mortality rates from breast cancer are in Spain, Norway, Finland and Portugal (below 20 deaths per 100 000 females), while the highest mortality rates are in Ireland and Denmark (above 30) (Figure 1.5.3).

Prostate cancer has become the most commonly occurring cancer among men in many EU countries, particularly for those aged over 65 years of age, although death rates from prostate cancer remain lower than for lung cancer in all countries except Sweden. The rise in the reported incidence of prostate cancer in many countries during the 1990s and 2000s was largely due to the greater use of prostate-specific antigen (PSA) diagnostic tests. Death rates from prostate cancer in 2008 varied from lows of less than 15 per 100 000 males in Malta and Romania, to highs of more than 30 per 100 000 males in a range of central and eastern European and Nordic countries (Figure 1.5.4). The causes of prostate cancer are not well-understood. Some evidence suggests that environmental and dietary factors might influence the risk of prostate cancer (Institute of Cancer Research, 2009).

Death rates from all types of cancer for males and females have declined at least slightly in most EU countries since 1994, although the decline has been more modest than for cardiovascular diseases, explaining why cancer accounts now for a larger share of all deaths. The exceptions to this declining pattern are among central and eastern European countries (Bulgaria, Romania, Latvia, Lithuania, Poland) and Greece, where cancer mortality has remained static or increased between 1994 and 2008.

Definition and deviations

Mortality rates are based on numbers of deaths registered in a country in a year divided by the size of the corresponding population. The rates have been directly age-standardised to the WHO European standard population to remove variations arising from differences in age structures across countries and over time. The source is the Eurostat Statistics Database.

The international comparability of cancer mortality data can be affected by differences in medical training and practices as well as in death certification procedures across countries. Mathers et al. (2005) have provided a general assessment of the coverage, completeness and reliability of data on causes of death.

Deaths from all cancers are classified to ICD-10 codes C00-C97, lung cancer to C32-C34, breast cancer to C50 and prostate cancer to C61.

1.5.1. All cancers mortality rates, males and females, 2008 (or nearest year available)

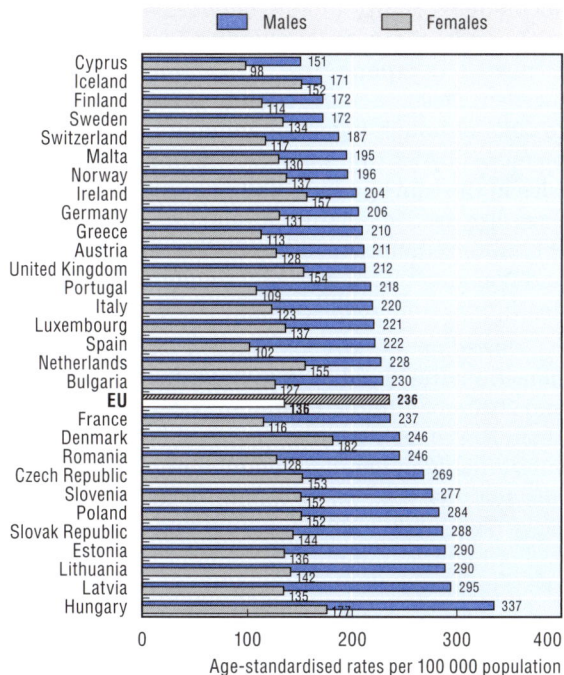

Source: Eurostat Statistics Database. Data are age-standardised to the WHO European standard population.

StatLink http://dx.doi.org/10.1787/888932335628

1.5.2. Lung cancer mortality rates, males and females, 2008 (or nearest year available)

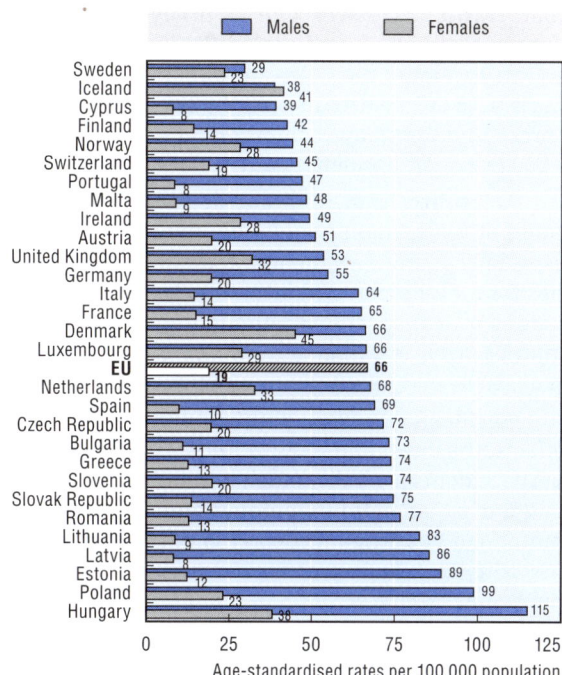

Source: Eurostat Statistics Database. Data are age-standardised to the WHO European standard population.

StatLink http://dx.doi.org/10.1787/888932335647

1.5.3. Breast cancer mortality rates, females, 2008 (or nearest year available)

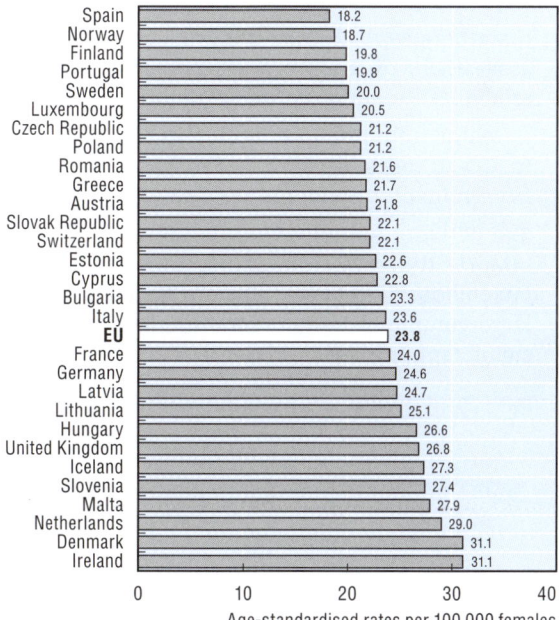

Source: Eurostat Statistics Database. Data are age-standardised to the WHO European standard population.

StatLink http://dx.doi.org/10.1787/888932335666

1.5.4. Prostate cancer mortality rates, males, 2008 (or nearest year available)

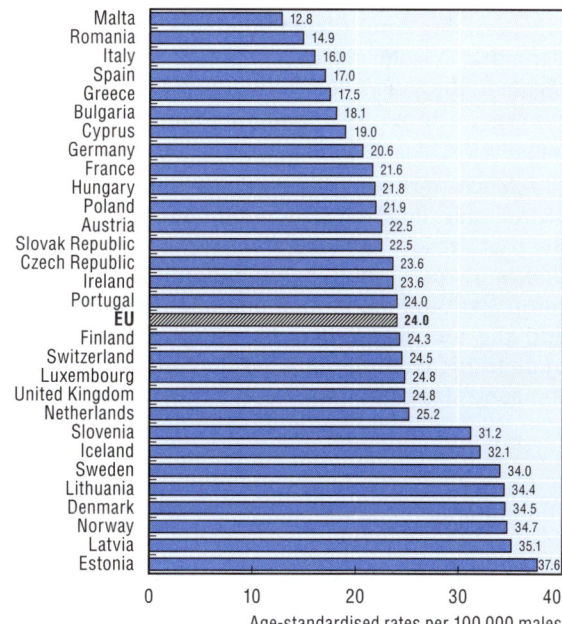

Source: Eurostat Statistics Database. Data are age-standardised to the WHO European standard population.

StatLink http://dx.doi.org/10.1787/888932335685

Worldwide, an estimated 1.2 million people are killed in transport accidents each year, mostly due to road traffic accidents, and as many as 50 million people are injured or disabled (WHO, 2009b). In EU countries alone, they were responsible for approximately 48 000 deaths in 2008. In 2008, Italy, Poland, France and Germany each experienced around 5 000-6 000 transport accident deaths.

Mortality from road accidents is the leading cause of death among children and young people, and especially young men, in many countries. The fatality risk for motor cycles and mopeds is highest among all modes of transport, even though most fatal traffic injuries occur in passenger vehicles (ETSC, 2003; Beck et al., 2007).

Besides the social, physical and psychological effects, the direct and indirect financial costs of transport accidents are substantial; one estimate put these at 2% of gross national product annually in highly-motorised countries (Peden et al., 2004). Injury and mortality from transport accidents remains a serious public health concern.

Death rates were the highest in 2008 in Lithuania, Romania and Latvia, all in excess of 15 deaths per 100 000 population (Figure 1.6.1). They were the lowest in Malta, the Netherlands, Iceland, Sweden and Switzerland, at five deaths per 100 000 population or less. A four-fold difference exists between the countries with the lowest and highest rates. Deaths from transport accidents are much higher for males than for females in all EU countries, with disparities in rates ranging from three times higher for males in Denmark, Sweden and Germany to five or more times higher in the Slovak Republic, Slovenia and Poland. On average, almost four times as many males than females die in transport accidents (Figure 1.6.1).

Much transport accident injury and mortality is preventable. Road security has increased greatly over the past decades in many countries through improvements of road systems, education and prevention campaigns, the adoption of new laws and regulations and the enforcement of these new laws through more traffic controls. As a result, death rates due to transport accidents have been cut by around 40% in EU countries since 1994 (Figures 1.6.2 and 1.6.3). Estonia has seen the largest decline in transport accident mortality of 78% between 1994 and 2008, with most of the fall occurring in the mid-1990s following independence. Reductions in Portugal, Sweden, Slovenia and Germany since 1994 are close to 60%, although vehicle kilometers travelled have increased by 2.7 times on average in European countries in the same period (OECD/ITF, 2008). Death rates have also declined in Greece, but at a slower pace, and therefore remain above the EU average. In Bulgaria and Romania there have been significant increases in death rates from road accidents since 1994.

Based on an extrapolation of past trends, projections from the World Bank indicate that between 2000 and 2020, road traffic deaths may decline further by about 30% in high-income countries, but may increase substantially in low- and middle-income countries if no additional road safety counter-measures are put in place (Peden et al., 2004).

Definition and deviations

Mortality rates are based on numbers of deaths registered in a country in a year divided by the size of the corresponding population. The rates have been directly age-standardised to the WHO European standard population to remove variations arising from differences in age structures across countries and over time. The source is the Eurostat Statistics Database.

Mathers et al. (2005) have provided a general assessment of the coverage, completeness and reliability of data on causes of death.

Deaths from transport accidents are classified to ICD-10 codes V01-V99. The majority of deaths from transport accidents are due to road traffic accidents.

Mortality rates from transport accidents in Luxembourg are biased upward because of the large volume of traffic in transit, resulting in a significant proportion of non-residents killed.

1.6.1. Transport accident mortality rates, 2008 (or nearest year available)

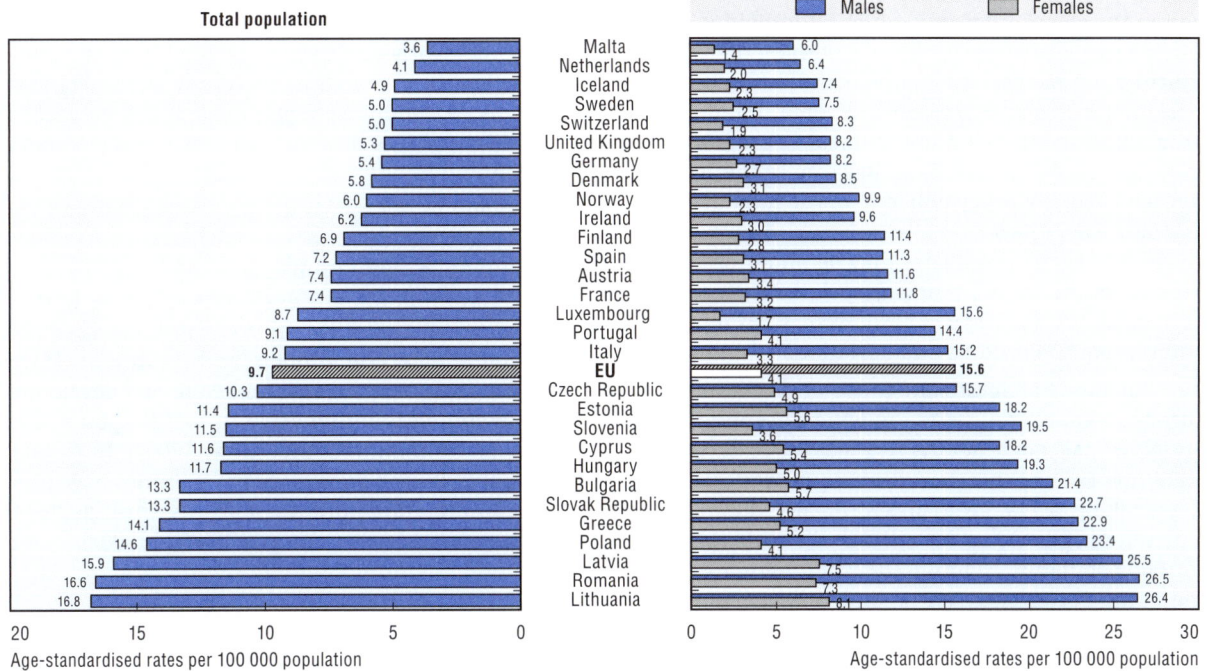

Source: Eurostat Statistics Database. Data are age-standardised to the WHO European standard population.

StatLink ᵐˢ⁴ http://dx.doi.org/10.1787/888932335704

1.6.2. Trends in transport accident mortality rates, selected EU countries, 1994-2008

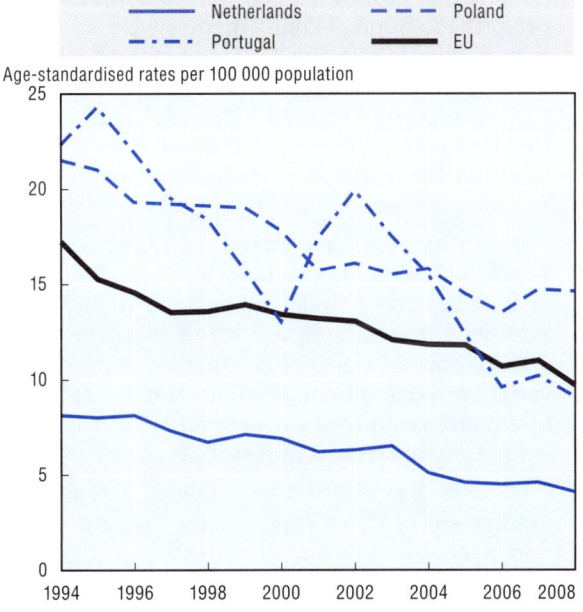

Source: Eurostat Statistics Database. Data are age-standardised to the WHO European standard population.

StatLink ᵐˢ⁴ http://dx.doi.org/10.1787/888932335723

1.6.3. Change in transport accident mortality rates, 1994-2008 (or nearest year available)

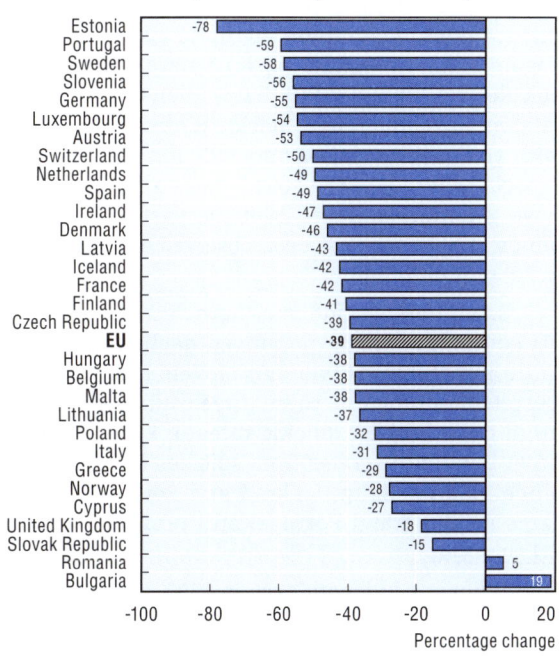

Source: Eurostat Statistics Database. Data are age-standardised to the WHO European standard population.

StatLink ᵐˢ⁴ http://dx.doi.org/10.1787/888932335742

The intentional killing of oneself is evidence not only of personal breakdown, but also of a deterioration of the social context in which an individual lives. Suicide may be the end-point of a number of different contributing factors. It is more likely to occur during crisis periods associated with divorce, alcohol and drug abuse, unemployment, clinical depression and other forms of mental illness. Because of this, suicide is often used as a proxy indicator of the mental health status of a population. However, the number of suicides in certain countries may be under-estimated because of the stigma that is associated with the act, or because of data issues associated with reporting criteria (see "Definitions and deviations").

Suicide is a significant cause of death in many European Union countries, and there were approximately 55 000 such deaths in 2008. Rates of suicide were low in southern European countries – Greece, Cyprus, Italy, Malta, Spain and Portugal – as well as the United Kingdom, at less than eight deaths per 100 000 population (Figure 1.7.1). They were highest in the Baltic States and Central and Eastern Europe; in Lithuania, Hungary and Latvia, as well as Finland, there were more than 18 deaths per 100 000 population. There is more than a ten-fold difference between Lithuania and Greece, the countries with the lowest and high death rates.

In general, death rates from suicides are three-to-four times greater for men than for women across the European Union, except in those countries with the highest rates, where rates are up to six times greater (Figure 1.7.1). The gender gap is narrower for attempted suicides, reflecting the fact that women tend to use less fatal methods than men. Suicide is also related to age, with young people aged under 25 and elderly people especially at risk. While suicide rates among the latter have generally declined over the past two decades, almost no progress has been observed among younger people.

Since 1994, suicide rates have decreased in many EU countries, with pronounced declines of 40% or more in Estonia, Latvia and Slovenia (Figure 1.7.2). Despite this progress, these three countries still have among the highest suicide rates in Europe. On the other hand, death rates from suicides have increased since 1994 in Malta, Iceland and Portugal, though rates in Malta and Portugal still remain below the EU average.

Following independence in 1990, suicide rates in Lithuania increased steadily, especially among young men, peaking in 1996 (Figure 1.7.3). The high suicide rates in Lithuania have been associated with a wide range of factors including rapid socio-economic transition, increasing psychological and social insecurity and the absence of a national suicide prevention strategy. Similarly in Hungary, societal factors including employment and socio-economic circumstances, as well as individual demographic and clinical factors have been cited as determinants of suicide (Almasi *et al.*, 2009).

Suicide is often linked with depression and the abuse of alcohol and other substances. Early detection of these psycho-social problems in high-risk groups by families and health professionals must be part of suicide prevention campaigns, together with the provision of effective support and treatment. Many countries are promoting mental health and developing national strategies for prevention, focusing on at-risk groups (Hawton and van Heeringen, 2009). In Finland and Iceland, suicide prevention programmes have been based on efforts to promote strong multisectoral collaboration and networking (NOMESCO, 2007).

Definition and deviations

The World Health Organization defines "suicide" as an act deliberately initiated and performed by a person in the full knowledge or expectation of its fatal outcome. Comparability of suicide data between countries is affected by a number of reporting criteria, including how a person's intention of killing themselves is ascertained, who is responsible for completing the death certificate, whether a forensic investigation is carried out, and the provisions for confidentiality of the cause of death. Caution is required therefore in interpreting variations across countries.

Mortality rates are based on numbers of deaths registered in a country in a year divided by the size of the corresponding population. The rates have been directly age-standardised to the WHO European standard population to remove variations arising from differences in age structures across countries and over time. The source is the *Eurostat Statistics Database*.

Mathers *et al.* (2005) have provided a general assessment of the coverage, completeness and reliability of data on causes of death.

Deaths from suicide are classified to ICD-10 codes X60-X84.

1.7.1. Suicide mortality rates, 2008 (or nearest year available)

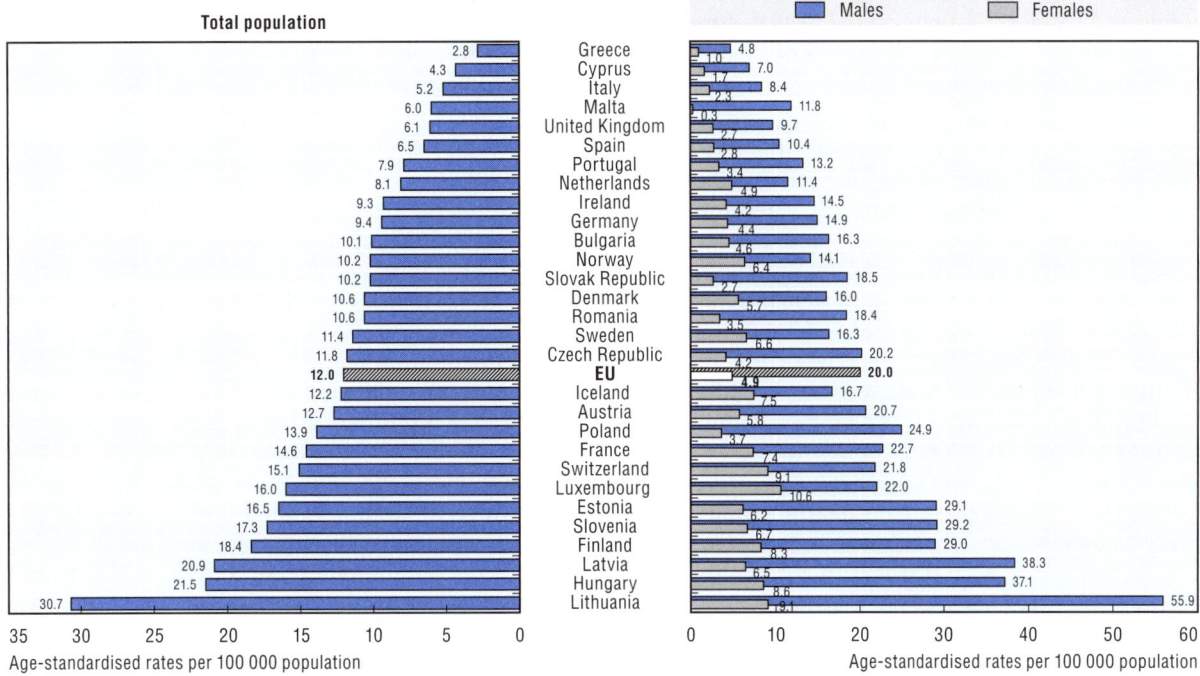

Source: Eurostat Statistics Database. Data are age-standardised to the WHO European standard population.

StatLink ⬛ http://dx.doi.org/10.1787/888932335761

1.7.2. Change in suicide rates, 1994-2008 (or nearest year available)

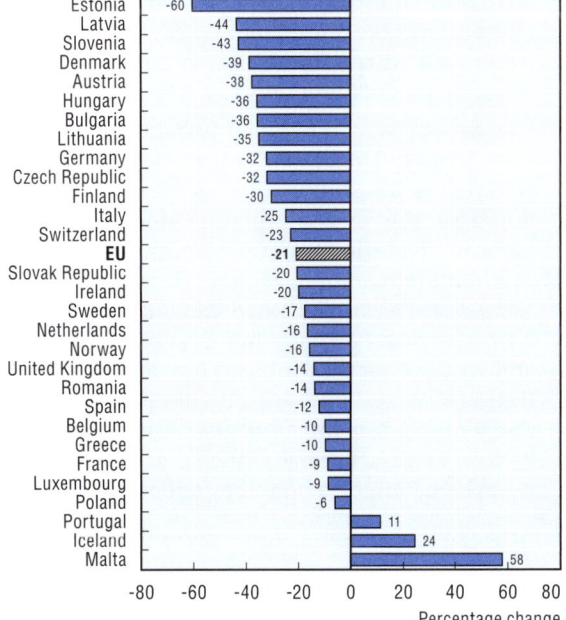

Source: Eurostat Statistics Database. Data are age-standardised to the WHO European standard population.

StatLink ⬛ http://dx.doi.org/10.1787/888932335780

1.7.3. Trends in suicide rates, selected EU countries, 1994-2008

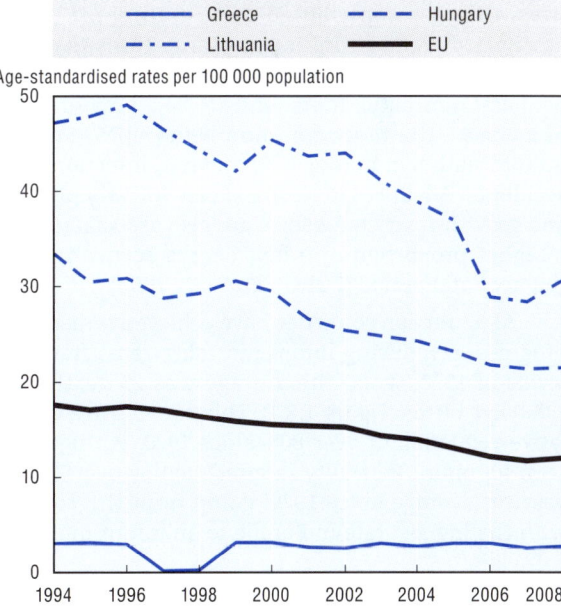

Source: Eurostat Statistics Database. Data are age-standardised to the WHO European standard population.

StatLink ⬛ http://dx.doi.org/10.1787/888932335799

Infant mortality, the rate at which babies of less than one year of age die, reflects the effect of economic and social conditions on the health of mothers and newborns, as well as the quality of medical care and preventive services.

In 2008, infant mortality rates in European countries ranged from a low of less than three deaths per 1 000 live births in Luxembourg, Slovenia, Nordic countries (with the exception of Denmark), Greece and the Czech Republic, up to a high of 11 and 17 deaths per 1 000 live births in Romania and Turkey respectively (Figure 1.8.1). Infant mortality rates were also relatively high (more than six deaths per 1 000 live births) in Latvia, Bulgaria and Malta. The average across the 27 European Union countries in 2008 was 4.6 deaths per 1 000 live births. Infant mortality rates tend to be higher than the EU average in central and eastern European countries, with the exceptions of Slovenia and the Czech Republic, both of which have had consistently lower rates.

Around two-thirds of the deaths that occur during the first year of life are neonatal deaths (i.e. during the first four weeks). Birth defects, prematurity and other conditions arising during pregnancy are the principal factors contributing to neonatal mortality in developed countries. With an increasing number of women deferring childbearing and the rise in multiple births linked with fertility treatments, the number of pre-term births has tended to increase (see Indicator 1.9). In a number of higher-income countries, this has contributed to a leveling-off of the downward trend in infant mortality rates over the past few years. For deaths beyond a month (post neonatal mortality), there tends to be a greater range of causes – the most common being SIDS (Sudden Infant Death Syndrome), birth defects, infections and accidents. Advances in neonatal care for very preterm and growth-restricted babies are also associated with a higher proportion of infant deaths occurring after the neonatal period (EURO-PERISTAT, 2008).

All European countries have achieved remarkable progress in reducing infant mortality rates from the levels of 1970, when the average was 25 deaths per 1 000 live births (Figure 1.8.1). This equates to a cumulative reduction of over 80% since 1970. Portugal has seen its infant mortality rate reduced by over 7% per year on average since 1970, going from the country with the highest rate in Europe to an infant mortality rate among the lowest in Europe in 2008 (Figure 1.8.2). Large reductions in infant mortality rates have also been observed in Luxembourg, Slovenia and Greece. On the other hand, the reduction in infant mortality rates has been slower in Latvia, Malta, Bulgaria and the Netherlands. Infant mortality rates in Poland declined rapidly in the early 1990s to approach the EU average.

Numerous studies have used infant mortality rates as a health outcome to examine the effect of a variety of medical and non-medical determinants of health (e.g. Joumard et al., 2008). Although most analyses show an overall negative relationship between infant mortality and health spending, the fact that some countries with a high level of health expenditure do not necessarily exhibit low levels of infant mortality has led some researchers to conclude that more health spending is not necessarily required to obtain better results (Retzlaff-Roberts et al., 2004). A body of research also suggests that many factors beyond the quality and efficiency of the health system, such as income inequality, the social environment, and individual lifestyles and attitudes, influence infant mortality rates (Kiely et al., 1995).

Definition and deviations

The infant mortality rate is the number of deaths of children under one year of age in a given year, expressed per 1 000 live births. Neonatal mortality refers to the death of children under 28 days.

Some of the international variation in infant and neonatal mortality rates may be due to variations among countries in registering practices of premature infants. Most countries have no gestational age or weight limits for mortality registration. Minimal limits exist for Norway (to be counted as a death following a live birth, the gestational age must exceed 12 weeks) and in the Czech Republic, France, Malta (the National Mortality Register), the Netherlands and Poland a minimum gestational age of 22 weeks and/or a weight threshold of 500 grams is applied. Lithuania has a gestational age limit.

1.8.1. Infant mortality rates, 2008 and decline 1970-2008

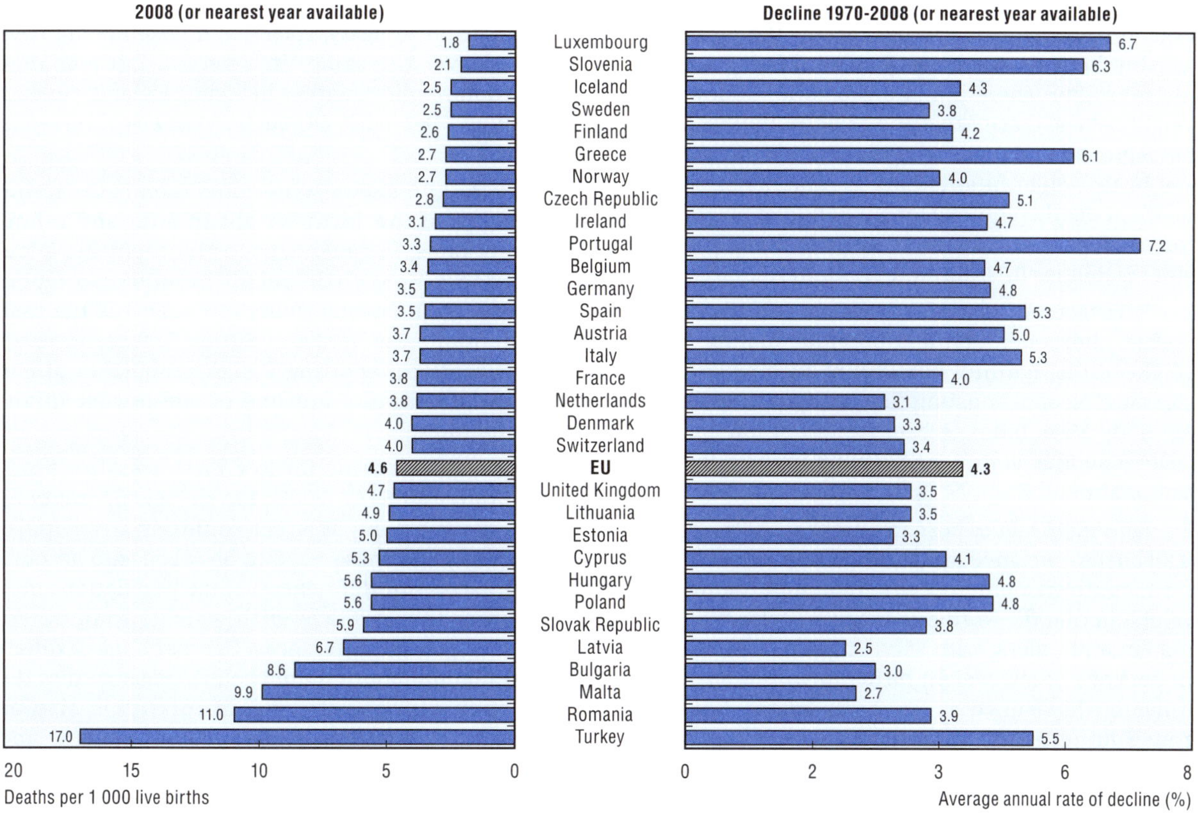

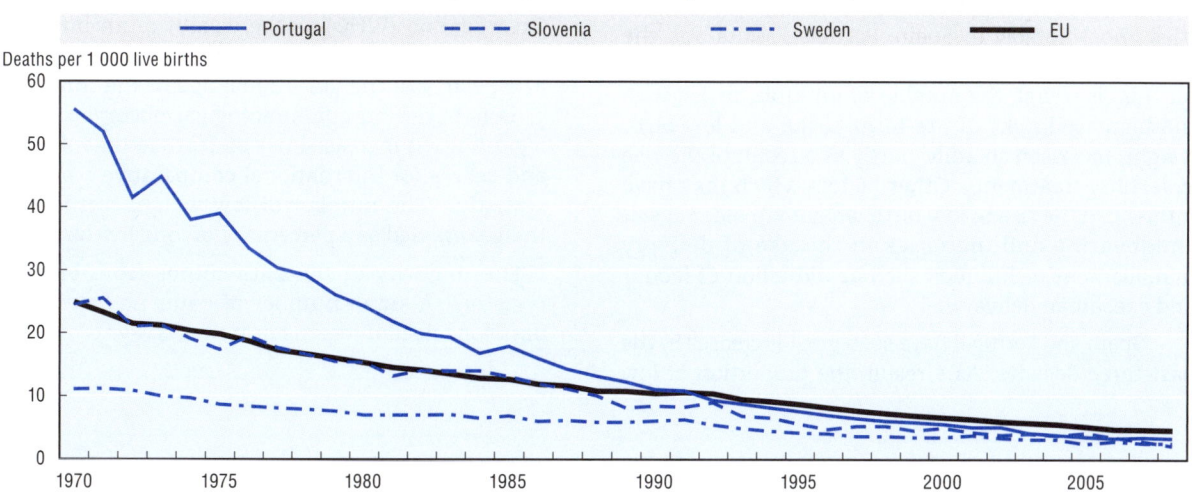

2008 (or nearest year available)
Decline 1970-2008 (or nearest year available)
Luxembourg 1.8 6.7
Slovenia 2.1 6.3
Iceland 2.5 4.3
Sweden 2.5 3.8
Finland 2.6 4.2
Greece 2.7 6.1
Norway 2.7 4.0
Czech Republic 2.8 5.1
Ireland 3.1 4.7
Portugal 3.3 7.2
Belgium 3.4 4.7
Germany 3.5 4.8
Spain 3.5 5.3
Austria 3.7 5.0
Italy 3.7 5.3
France 3.8 4.0
Netherlands 3.8 3.1
Denmark 4.0 3.3
Switzerland 4.0 3.4
EU 4.6 4.3
United Kingdom 4.7 3.5
Lithuania 4.9 3.5
Estonia 5.0 3.3
Cyprus 5.3 4.1
Hungary 5.6 4.8
Poland 5.6 4.8
Slovak Republic 5.9 3.8
Latvia 6.7 2.5
Bulgaria 8.6 3.0
Malta 9.9 2.7
Romania 11.0 3.9
Turkey 17.0 5.5
20
15
10
5
0
Deaths per 1 000 live births
0
2
3
6
8
Average annual rate of decline (%)

Source: *OECD Health Data 2010; Eurostat Statistics Database.*

StatLink http://dx.doi.org/10.1787/888932335818

1.8.2. Infant mortality rates, selected European countries, 1970-2008

Portugal
Slovenia
Sweden
EU
Deaths per 1 000 live births
60
50
40
30
20
10
0
1970
1975
1980
1985
1990
1995
2000
2005

Source: *OECD Health Data 2010; Eurostat Statistics Database.*

StatLink http://dx.doi.org/10.1787/888932335837

Low birth weight – defined here as newborns weighing less than 2 500 grams – is an important indicator of infant health because of the close relationship between birth weight and infant morbidity and mortality. There are two categories of low birth weight babies: those occurring as a result of restricted foetal growth and those resulting from pre-term birth. Low birth weight infants have a greater risk of poor health or death, require a longer period of hospitalisation after birth, and are more likely to develop significant disabilities (UNICEF and WHO, 2004).

Risk factors for low birth weight include adolescent motherhood, having a previous history of low weight births, harmful behaviours such as smoking, excessive alcohol consumption and poor nutrition, a low Body Mass Index, a background of low parental socio-economic status, and having in-vitro fertilisation treatment.

One-in-16 babies born in Europe in 2008 – or 6.4% of all births – weighed less than 2 500 grams at birth. A north-south gradient is evident in Europe for low birth weight, in that the Nordic countries – Iceland, Sweden and Finland – along with Latvia reported the smallest proportions of low weight births, with less than 4.5% of live births defined as low birth weight. Countries from Southern Europe including Greece, Spain and Portugal, as well as Turkey, Romania, Bulgaria and Hungary, are at the other end of the scale with rates of low birth weight infants above 7.5%. The proportion of low birth weight among European countries varies by a factor of more than two (Figure 1.9.1).

Since 1980 the prevalence of low birth weight infants has increased in a number of European countries, most notably in Spain, Portugal, Malta and the Netherlands (Figure 1.9.1). There are several reasons for this rise. First, the number of multiple births, with the increased risks of pre-term births and low birth weight, has risen steadily, partly as a result of the rise in fertility treatments. Other factors which may have influenced the rise in low birth weight are older age at childbearing and increases in the use of delivery management techniques such as induction of labour and caesarean delivery.

Spain and Portugal have seen great increases in the past three decades. As a result, the proportion of low birth weight babies in these countries is now above the European average (Figure 1.9.2). Low birth weight proportions in Hungary, Poland and Luxembourg have declined over the same time period. Little change occurred in Nordic countries including Iceland, Finland, Sweden and Denmark, although a rise was observed in Norway.

Figure 1.9.3 shows some correlation between the percentage of low birth weight infants and infant mortality rates. In general, countries reporting a low proportion of low birth weight infants also report relatively low infant mortality rates. This is the case for instance for the Nordic countries. Greece, however, is an exception, reporting a high proportion of low birth weight infants but one of the lowest infant mortality rates.

Agreed-on norms for low birth weight do not exist (EURO-PERISTAT, 2008). Physiological variations in size occur among different countries and population groups, and these need to be taken into account when interpreting differences. Some populations may have lower than average birth weights than others because of genetic differences. Comparisons of different population groups within countries show that the proportion of low birth weight infants is also be influenced by differences in education, income and associated living conditions.

Definition and deviations

Low birth weight is defined by the World Health Organization (WHO) as the weight of an infant at birth of less than 2 500 grams (5.5 pounds), irrespective of the gestational age of the infant. This is based on epidemiological observations regarding the increased risk of death to the infant and serves for international comparative health statistics. The number of low weight births is then expressed as a percentage of total live births.

The majority of the data comes from birth registers. A small number of countries supply data for selected regions or from surveys.

1.9.1. Low birth weight infants, 2008 and change 1980-2008

2008 (or nearest year available)

Country	%
Iceland	3.8
Finland	4.1
Sweden	4.1
Latvia	4.3
Estonia	4.6
Lithuania	4.6
Luxembourg	4.6
Norway	5.1
Ireland	5.3
Poland	5.7
Denmark	5.8
Netherlands	6.2
Slovenia	6.3
Switzerland	6.3
EU	**6.4**
Italy	6.7
Malta	6.8
France	6.8
Germany	6.8
Austria	7.1
United Kingdom	7.1
Czech Republic	7.3
Slovak Republic	7.3
Belgium	7.6
Spain	7.6
Portugal	7.7
Romania	7.9
Bulgaria	8.3
Hungary	8.3
Greece	8.4
Turkey	11.0

Percentage of newborns weighing less than 2 500 g

Change 1980-2008 (or nearest year available)

Country	% change
Iceland	12
Finland	5
Sweden	-2
Latvia	n.a.
Estonia	n.a.
Lithuania	n.a.
Luxembourg	-27
Norway	34
Ireland	33
Poland	-25
Denmark	0
Netherlands	55
Slovenia	9
Switzerland	24
EU	**15**
Italy	20
Malta	62
France	31
Germany	24
Austria	25
United Kingdom	6
Czech Republic	24
Slovak Republic	24
Belgium	36
Spain	171
Portugal	67
Romania	4
Bulgaria	36
Hungary	-20
Greece	42
Turkey	n.a.

% change over period

Source: OECD Health Data 2010; WHO HFA-DB.

StatLink http://dx.doi.org/10.1787/888932335856

1.9.2. Trends in low birth weight infants, selected European countries, 1980-2008

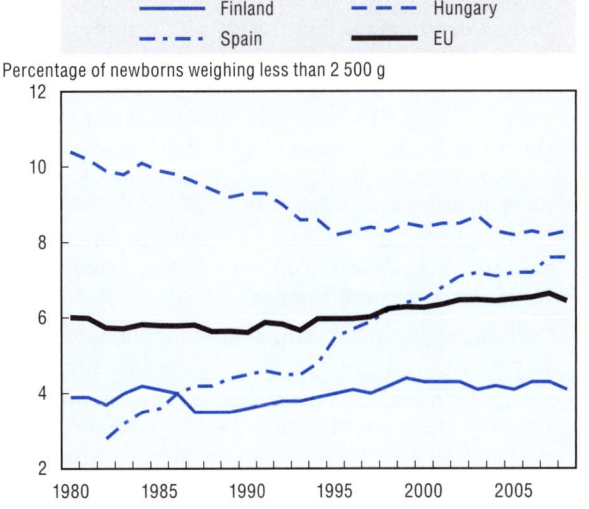

Legend: Finland, Hungary, Spain, EU

Percentage of newborns weighing less than 2 500 g

Source: OECD Health Data 2010; WHO HFA-DB.
StatLink http://dx.doi.org/10.1787/888932335875

1.9.3. Low birth weight and infant mortality, 2008 (or nearest year available)

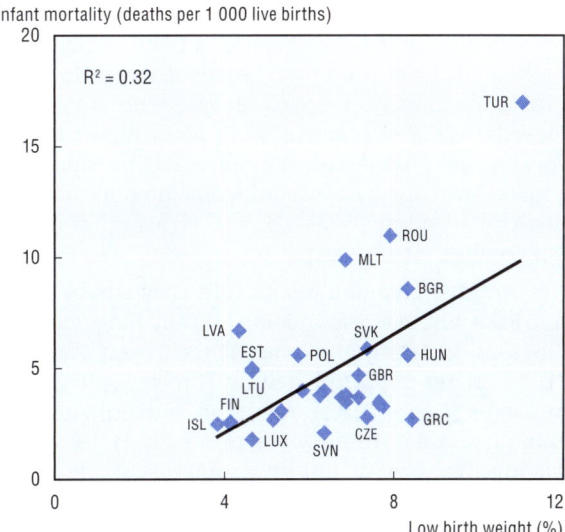

Infant mortality (deaths per 1 000 live births)

$R^2 = 0.32$

Low birth weight (%)

Source: OECD Health Data 2010; WHO HFA-DB.
StatLink http://dx.doi.org/10.1787/888932335894

Most European countries conduct regular health surveys which allow respondents to report on different aspects of their health. A commonly-asked question relates to self-perceived health status, of the type: "How is your health in general?". Despite the subjective nature of this question, indicators of perceived general health have been found to be a good predictor of people's future health care use and mortality (for instance, see Miilunpalo et al., 1997). For the purpose of international comparisons however, cross-country differences in perceived health status are difficult to interpret because responses may be affected by social and cultural factors.

Keeping these limitations in mind, a majority of the adult population in almost all European countries rate their health to be good or very good (Figure 1.10.1). In Switzerland, Ireland, Iceland and the United Kingdom, more than eight out of ten people report good or very good health. Across the European Union, two-thirds (67%) of all adults rated their health as good or better, with Germany, Finland and France close to this average. Adults in central and eastern European countries, along with Portugal, report the lowest rates of good or very good health. In Latvia, Lithuania and Portugal, less than half of all adults consider themselves to be in good health. These differences, however, do not necessarily mean that the general health of people in Switzerland or Ireland is objectively better than that of citizens in Latvia or Portugal (Baert and de Norre, 2009).

In all European countries, men are more likely than women to rate their health as good or better, with the largest differences in Portugal, Bulgaria and the Slovak Republic. Unsurprisingly, people's rating of their own health tends to decline with age. In many countries there is a particularly marked decline in a positive rating of one's own health after age 45 and a further decline after age 65. People who are unemployed, retired or inactive more often report bad or very bad health (Baert and de Norre, 2009). People with a lower level of education or income do not rate their health as positively as people with higher levels (Mackenbach et al., 2008).

Another common health interview survey question asks whether respondents had any long-standing illnesses or health problems. Three-in-ten adults in EU countries reported having illnesses or health problems (Figure 1.10.1). Adults in Finland, Slovenia, Hungary and Estonia were more likely to report having illnesses or health problems, while these conditions were less commonly reported in Romania, Greece and Italy. Women reported long-standing illnesses or health problems more often than men (an average of 32% versus 27% across EU countries), with the gender divide greatest in Latvia, Norway and the Slovak Republic. Reporting increased with age, from an average of 10% of young people aged 15-24 years, to 70% of older persons aged 85 years or more. There is a moderate negative association between adults reporting good/very good health, and reporting a long-standing illness or health problem ($R^2 = -0.38$).

When adults were asked whether they had been limited in their usual daily activities because of a health problem – which is one definition of disability – 24% answered that they had, with 8% of respondents "strongly limited" and 15% "limited to some extent" (Figure 1.10.2). Adults most commonly reported activity limitation in the Slovak Republic, Germany, Latvia, Estonia and Portugal (30% or more of respondents), and less so in Malta, Iceland and Switzerland (less than 15%). Severe activity limitation was more prevalent in Portugal, the Slovak Republic, Austria and Germany (10% or more of respondents), and less so in Malta, Bulgaria and Switzerland (less than 5%). Adults with activity limitations were also less likely to report good or very good health ($R^2 = 0.60$).

1.10.1. Adults' self-reported health status, 2008

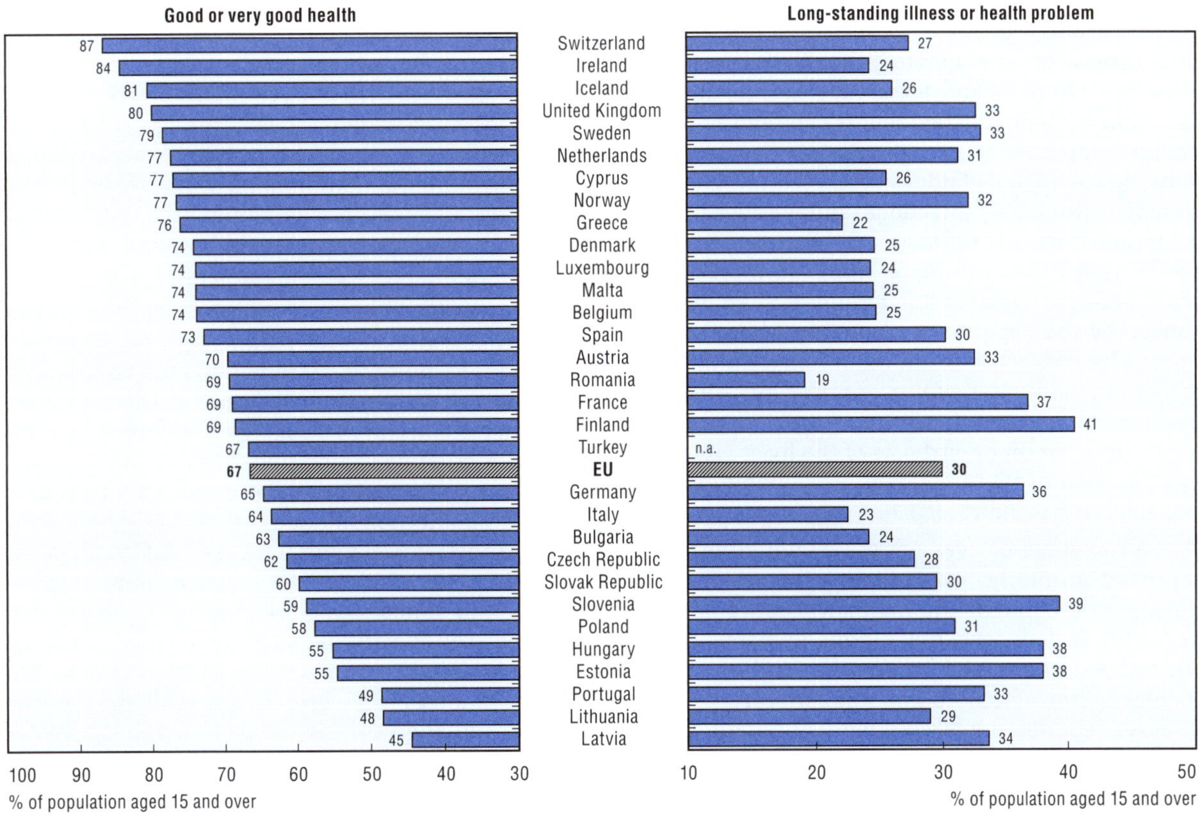

Good or very good health
Long-standing illness or health problem
Switzerland 87 27
Ireland 84 24
Iceland 81 26
United Kingdom 80 33
Sweden 79 33
Netherlands 77 31
Cyprus 77 26
Norway 77 32
Greece 76 22
Denmark 74 25
Luxembourg 74 24
Malta 74 25
Belgium 74 25
Spain 73 30
Austria 70 33
Romania 69 19
France 69 37
Finland 69 41
Turkey 67 n.a.
EU 67 30
Germany 65 36
Italy 64 23
Bulgaria 63 24
Czech Republic 62 28
Slovak Republic 60 30
Slovenia 59 39
Poland 58 31
Hungary 55 38
Estonia 55 38
Portugal 49 33
Lithuania 48 29
Latvia 45 34
100 90 80 70 60 50 40 30
10 20 30 40 50
% of population aged 15 and over
% of population aged 15 and over

Source: EU-Statistics on Income and Living Conditions survey; *OECD Health Data 2010*; Swiss Federal Statistics Office.

StatLink http://dx.doi.org/10.1787/888932335913

1.10.2. Adults reporting a limitation in usual activities, 2008

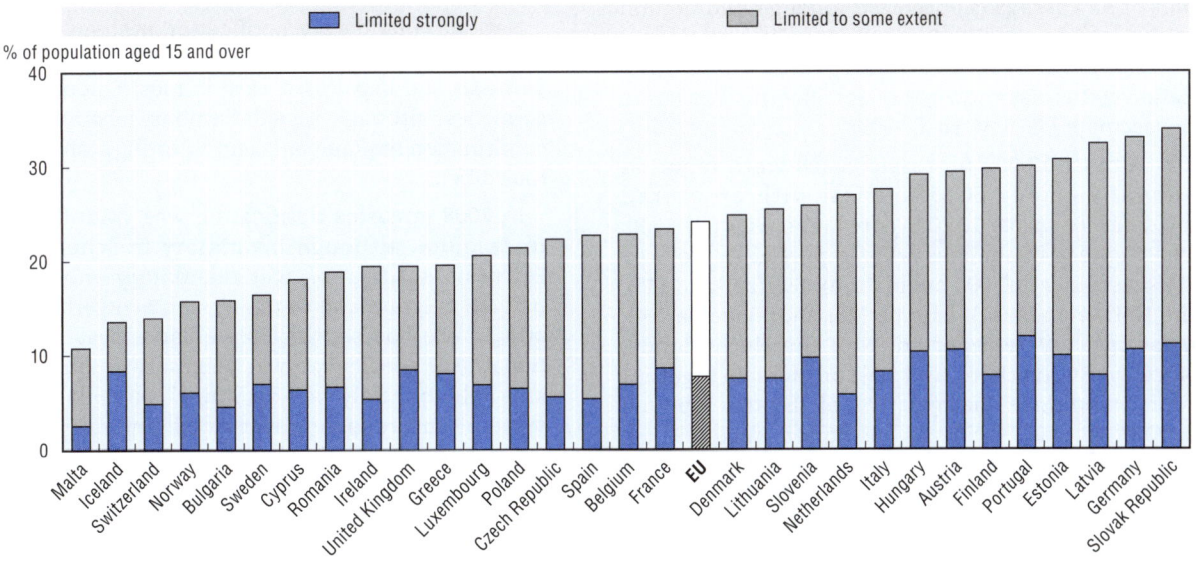

Limited strongly
Limited to some extent
% of population aged 15 and over
40
30
20
10
0
Malta
Iceland
Switzerland
Norway
Bulgaria
Sweden
Cyprus
Romania
Ireland
United Kingdom
Greece
Luxembourg
Poland
Czech Republic
Spain
Belgium
France
EU
Denmark
Lithuania
Slovenia
Netherlands
Italy
Hungary
Austria
Finland
Portugal
Estonia
Latvia
Germany
Slovak Republic

Source: EU-Statistics on Income and Living Conditions survey; Swiss Federal Statistics Office.

StatLink http://dx.doi.org/10.1787/888932335932

Communicable diseases such as measles, pertussis and hepatitis B still pose a major threat to the health of European citizens. Measles, a highly infectious disease of the respiratory system, is caused by a virus. Symptoms include fever, cough, runny nose, red eyes and a characteristic rash. It can lead to severe health complications, including pneumonia, encephalitis, diarrhoea and blindness. Pertussis (or whooping cough) is also highly infectious, and is caused by the bacterium *Bordetella pertussis*. The disease derives its name from the sound made from the intake of air after a cough. Hepatitis B is an infection of the liver caused by the hepatitis B virus. The virus is transmitted by contact with blood or body fluids of an infected person. A small proportion of infections become chronic, and these people are at high risk of death from cancer or cirrhosis of the liver. Protection against each of these diseases is available through vaccination (see Indicator 3.3).

An average of over 5 000 measles cases were reported annually in European Union countries during 2006-08, with the highest number of cases occurring in four countries: Germany, Romania, the United Kingdom and Italy. The highest crude incidence during 2006-08 was in Switzerland, with 15 cases reported per 100 000 persons (Figure 1.11.1). A number of other western European countries, including the United Kingdom, Romania, France and Italy, also had high incidences. Across the European Union, average incidence for 2006-08 was 1.2 cases per 100 000 population. This represents a marked decline from the average rate in 1991-93, which was 27 cases per 100 000 population. In 2008, more than half of all cases (53%) occurred among children and young people aged 5-19 years. Hospitalisation was necessary for 15% of cases. Among cases whose vaccination status was known, the vast majority (91%) were unvaccinated (EUVAC.NET, 2009).

Almost 13 000 pertussis cases were reported annually among EU countries, with an overall incidence of six per 100 000 population (Figure 1.11.2). The highest incidences were reported in Norway (113 cases per 100 000 population), Switzerland (45), the Netherlands (41), Estonia (26) and Slovenia (24). Most cases were reported from the Netherlands, Norway, Switzerland and Poland, which together contributed three-quarters (76%) of all cases reported in 2008. Pertussis incidence has halved since 1991-93, when the average rate among EU countries was 11.3 notified cases per 100 000 population.

Two-thirds of all pertussis cases in 2008 occurred among children aged under 15 years of age, although the disease may be under-diagnosed in adolescents and adults. The highest incidence occurred among infants aged less than one year, many of whom are too young to be vaccinated, and children aged 10-14 years, who may have not had a full course of vaccination, or who may have lost their immunity. Vaccination status was known in only half of all reported cases, but of these 21% were unvaccinated (EUVAC.NET, 2010).

Around 6 000 hepatitis B cases were reported annually in EU countries during 2006-08. The highest incidence rates occurred among six countries: Iceland (13.2 notified cases per 100 000 population), Bulgaria (9.9), Turkey (9.1), Austria (8.1), Latvia (7.3) and Romania (5.1) (Figure 1.11.3). The notification rate has declined in EU countries since 1991-93, when it was 8.3 cases per 100 000 population to 2.5 for 2006-08. Hepatitis B infection is more common in the southern parts of Eastern and Central Europe, and low in prevalence in most of Western Europe. Around twice as many cases of hepatitis B occurred among males than females in 2008, with the majority reported in the age group 25-44 years, followed by 15-24 year-olds. The disease is increasingly seen as a sexually transmitted disease, although the disease pattern and risk groups differ widely across Europe (ECDC, 2009).

Definition and deviations

National mandatory notification systems for communicable diseases, including measles, pertussis and hepatitis B, exist in most European countries, although case definitions, laboratory confirmation requirements and reporting systems may differ.

In 2008, measles notification was voluntary in Belgium, although mandatory in schools. Pertussis notification was mandatory only in parts of Belgium and Germany, and Switzerland and France had sentinel surveillance systems. Hepatitis B notification was voluntary in France and Belgium, Italy had a sentinel surveillance system, and reporting was not mandatory in Switzerland.

1.11.1. Incidence of measles, 2006-08

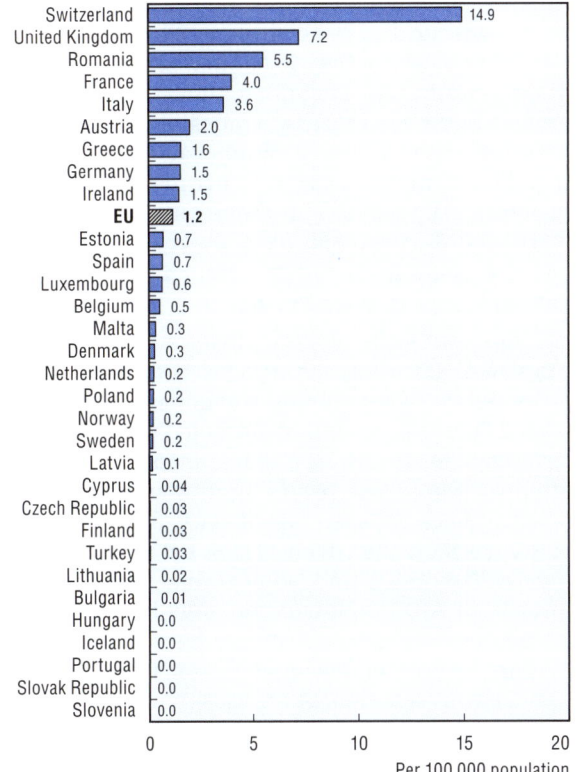

Source: OECD Health Data 2010; WHO Europe (2010).

StatLink http://dx.doi.org/10.1787/888932335951

1.11.2. Incidence of pertussis, 2006-08

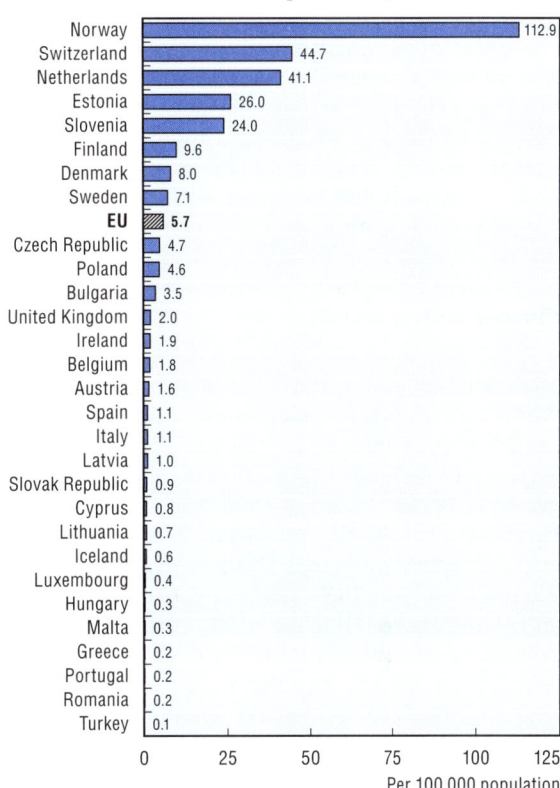

Source: OECD Health Data 2010; WHO Europe (2010).

StatLink http://dx.doi.org/10.1787/888932335970

1.11.3. Incidence of hepatitis B, 2006-08

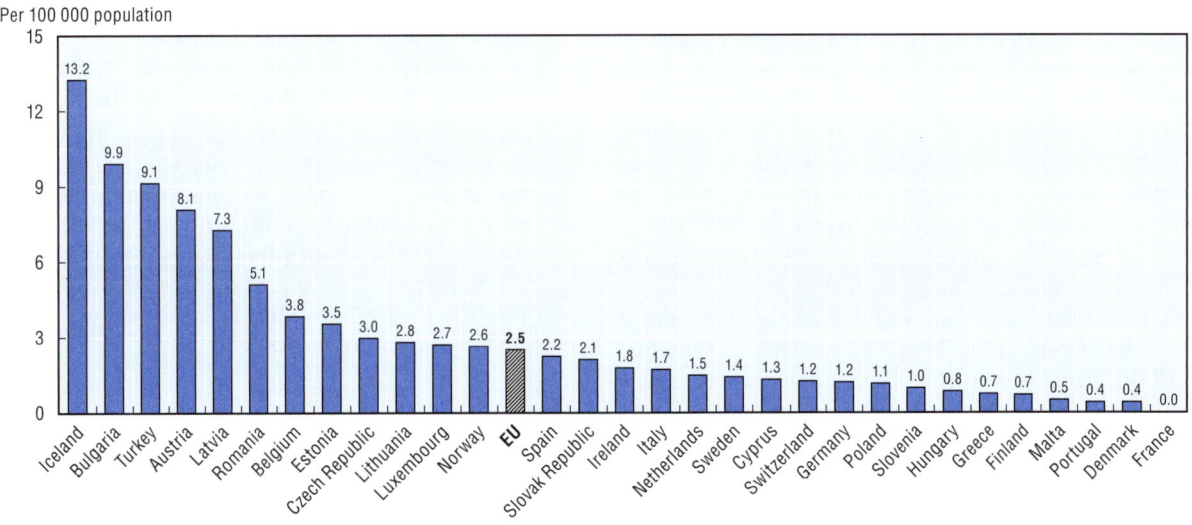

Source: OECD Health Data 2010; WHO Europe (2010).

StatLink http://dx.doi.org/10.1787/888932335989

The first cases of Acquired Immunodeficiency Syndrome (AIDS) were diagnosed almost 30 years ago. The onset of AIDS is normally caused as a result of HIV (human immunodeficiency virus) infection and can manifest itself as any number of different diseases, such as pneumonia and tuberculosis, as the immune system is no longer able to defend the body. There is a time lag between HIV infection, AIDS diagnosis and death due to HIV infection, which can be any number of years depending on the treatment administered. Despite worldwide research, there is no cure currently available.

In 2008, the number of newly reported cases of AIDS was approximately 5 300 across the European Union as a whole, representing an unweighted average incidence rate of 12.7 per million population (Figure 1.12.1). Following the first reporting of AIDS in the early 1980s, the number of cases rose rapidly to reach an average of more than 37 new cases per million population across EU countries at its peak in the middle of the 1990s, almost three times current incidence rates (Figure 1.12.2). Public awareness campaigns contributed to steady declines in reported cases through the second half of the 1990s. In addition, the development and greater availability of antiretroviral drugs, which reduce or slow down the development of the disease, led to a sharp decrease in incidence from 1996.

The highest AIDS incidence rates among EU countries in 2008 were reported in Estonia, Latvia, Portugal and Spain, at 25-50 new cases per million population. Spain had the highest incidence rates in the first decade following the outbreak, although there was a sharp decline from 1994 onwards. Incidence rates in Portugal peaked somewhat later, towards the end of the 1990s. AIDS incidence rates in Estonia have increased rapidly since the mid-2000s. Central European countries such as the Czech and Slovak Republics, Hungary and Poland report the lowest incidence rates of AIDS among EU countries.

In the European Union, approximately 730 000 persons were living with HIV infection in 2007 (Figure 1.12.1). Italy, Spain and France had the greatest number of persons, followed by the United Kingdom and Germany. HIV prevalence estimates were highest in those countries with high AIDS incidence rates – Estonia, Latvia, Portugal and Spain, along with Switzerland – all at over 300 persons per 100 000 population. Over 25 000 new cases of HIV were diagnosed in the European Union in 2008. The predominant mode of transmission of HIV is sex between men, followed by heterosexual contact. However, among eastern European countries, injecting drug use is still the most common mode (ECDC and WHO Europe, 2009). Approximately 75% of heterosexually acquired HIV infection in Western and Central Europe is among migrants.

In recent years, the overall decline in AIDS cases has slowed down. This reversal has been accompanied by evidence of increasing transmission of HIV in several European countries, attributed to complacency regarding the effectiveness of treatment and a waning of public awareness regarding drug use and sexual practice. Since 2000, the rate of newly diagnosed cases of HIV has more than doubled to 89 per million population in 2008 (ECDC and WHO Europe, 2009). Further inroads in AIDS incidence rates will require more intensive evidence-based HIV prevention programmes that are focused and adapted to reach those most at risk of HIV infection (UNAIDS, 2008).

Definition and deviations

The incidence rate of acquired immunodeficiency syndrome (AIDS) is the number of new cases per million population at year of diagnosis. Note that data for recent years are provisional due to reporting delays, which sometimes can be for several years depending on the country.

Estimates of the number of persons living with human Immunodeficiency virus (HIV) are calculated by the Joint United Nations Programme on HIV/AIDS (UNAIDS, 2008), and are based on national research studies. These estimates include all people (adults and children) with HIV infection in 2007, whether or not they have developed symptoms of AIDS.

1.12.1. AIDS incidence rates in 2008, and estimated number of persons living with HIV in 2007

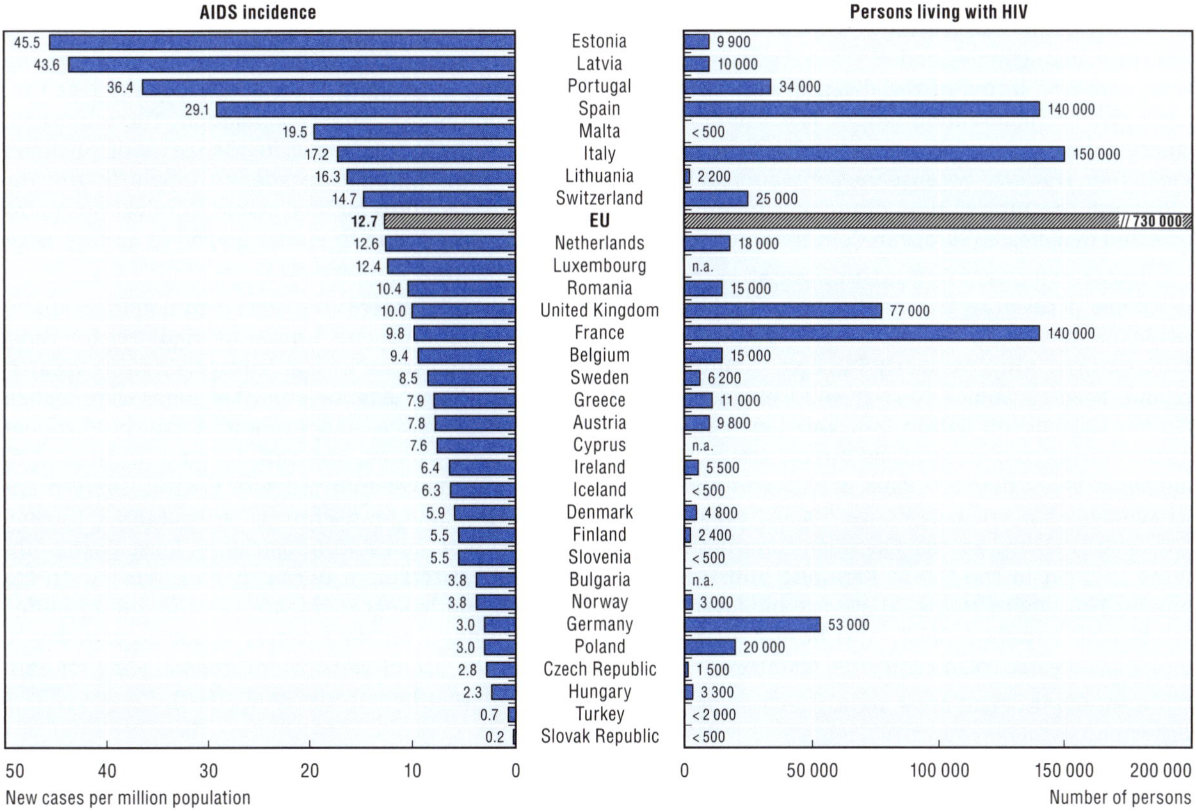

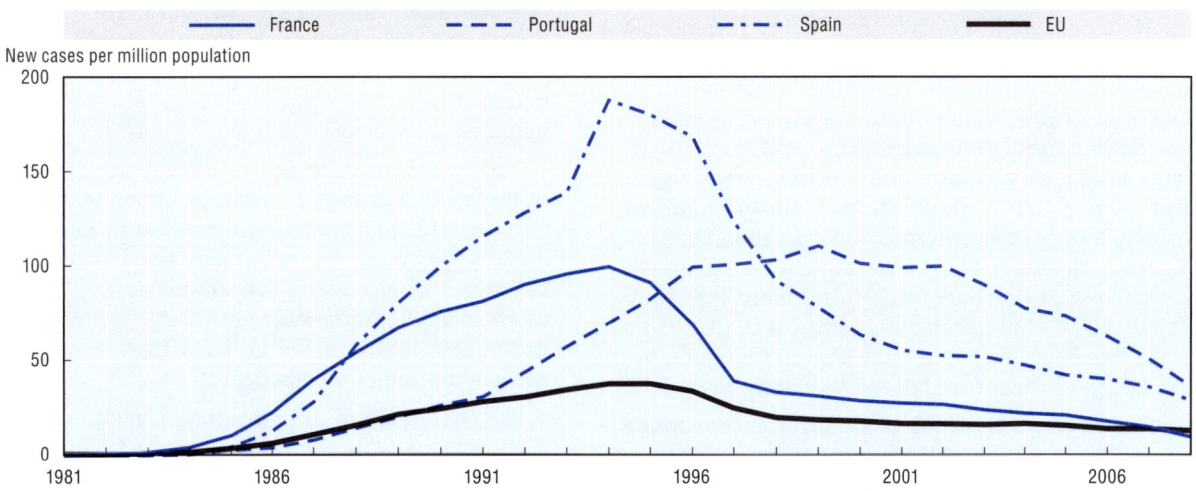

AIDS incidence

Country	New cases per million population
Estonia	45.5
Latvia	43.6
Portugal	36.4
Spain	29.1
Malta	19.5
Italy	17.2
Lithuania	16.3
Switzerland	14.7
EU	**12.7**
Netherlands	12.6
Luxembourg	12.4
Romania	10.4
United Kingdom	10.0
France	9.8
Belgium	9.4
Sweden	8.5
Greece	7.9
Austria	7.8
Cyprus	7.6
Ireland	6.4
Iceland	6.3
Denmark	5.9
Finland	5.5
Slovenia	5.5
Bulgaria	3.8
Norway	3.8
Germany	3.0
Poland	3.0
Czech Republic	2.8
Hungary	2.3
Turkey	0.7
Slovak Republic	0.2

Persons living with HIV

Country	Number of persons
Estonia	9 900
Latvia	10 000
Portugal	34 000
Spain	140 000
Malta	< 500
Italy	150 000
Lithuania	2 200
Switzerland	25 000
EU	**730 000**
Netherlands	18 000
Luxembourg	n.a.
Romania	15 000
United Kingdom	77 000
France	140 000
Belgium	15 000
Sweden	6 200
Greece	11 000
Austria	9 800
Cyprus	n.a.
Ireland	5 500
Iceland	< 500
Denmark	4 800
Finland	2 400
Slovenia	< 500
Bulgaria	n.a.
Norway	3 000
Germany	53 000
Poland	20 000
Czech Republic	1 500
Hungary	3 300
Turkey	< 2 000
Slovak Republic	< 500

Source: OECD Health Data 2010; ECDC and WHO Europe (2009); UNAIDS (2008).

StatLink ⟳ http://dx.doi.org/10.1787/888932336008

1.12.2. Trends in AIDS incidence rates, selected EU countries, 1981-2008

Legend: France — Portugal --- Spain -·-·- EU ▬

New cases per million population (y-axis: 0, 50, 100, 150, 200)

x-axis: 1981, 1986, 1991, 1996, 2001, 2006

Source: OECD Health Data 2010.

StatLink ⟳ http://dx.doi.org/10.1787/888932336027

Around 2.4 million new cases of cancer (excluding non-melanoma skin cancers) were diagnosed in EU countries in 2008 (Ferlay et al., 2010), with 55% occurring among males and 45% among females. The most common forms of the disease were prostate, colorectal, breast and lung cancer. The risk of getting cancer before the age of 75 years is 26.5%, or around one in four. However, because the population of Europe is ageing, the rate of new cases of cancer is also expected to increase (European Commission, 2008b).

Large regional inequalities exist in cancer incidence across the European Union. In 2008, the incidence rate for all cancers combined was highest in Northern and Western Europe – Denmark, Ireland, Belgium, France, Norway and Iceland – at over 290 per 100 000 population, but was lower in some Mediterranean countries such as Turkey, Greece, Cyprus and Malta, at less than 220. Rates in Italy were above the EU average of 255 new cases per 100 000 population. Rates in central and eastern European countries varied, being highest in the Czech Republic and Hungary (around 290), similar to the EU average in Slovenia and the Slovak Republic (260), and below average in Romania, Bulgaria, Poland and other countries.

Cancer incidence rates are higher for men than for women in all EU countries (Figure 1.13.1). Here too there is great variation between countries; in Spain and Turkey, male incidence rates are 60% higher than female rates, whereas in Denmark and Cyprus they are less than 10% higher. The average all cancer incidence rate among EU member states was 298 per 100 000 males and 226 per 100 000 females.

In 2008, lung cancer was one of the most common cancers in EU countries, being responsible for around 12% of all new cancer diagnoses, 16% for males and 7% for females. Ten of the fifteen countries with male rates higher than the EU average were located in Central and Eastern Europe (Figure 1.13.2). Rates in Hungary, Poland and Slovenia were higher than 60 per 100 000 population. Male lung cancer incidence rates in Northern Europe (Sweden, Iceland, Finland, Norway) and some southern European countries (Cyprus, Portugal, Malta) were less than 40 per 100 000 population. Among females, lung cancer incidence was especially high in Denmark, but also Hungary, Iceland and the Netherlands, at over 25.

Thirty per cent of all new cancer cases among women diagnosed in 2008 were cancers of the breast – the most common form of cancer among women. Incidence rates were high in western European countries such as Belgium, France, the Netherlands and Ireland, at over 90 cases per 100 000 population (Figure 1.13.3). Rates in Central, Eastern and Southern Europe were lower, with Turkey, Greece, Romania, Lithuania, Latvia and Poland all reporting less than 50 new cases per 100 000 population. There has been an increase in measured incidence rates of breast cancer over the past decade, although death rates have declined or remained stable. Survival rates have also increased, due to earlier diagnosis and/or better treatment (see Indicator 3.13).

Prostate cancer is the most common form among men in the European Union, particularly for those aged over 65 years of age, comprising one quarter (25%) of all new diagnoses in 2008. Rates were highest in Ireland, France, Belgium and northern European countries (Norway, Sweden, Iceland and Finland). Rates were lower in a range of central, eastern and southern European countries, including Turkey, Greece, Romania and Bulgaria. At least part of the five-fold difference between countries with the highest and lowest incidence rates is due to under-registration of prostate cancer in some countries, as well as the use of sensitive diagnostic tests for early detection in others (Ferlay et al., 2007).

Definition and deviations

Cancer incidence rates are based on numbers of new cases of cancer registered in a country in a year divided by the size of the corresponding population. The rates have been directly age-standardised to the WHO World standard population to remove variations arising from differences in age structures across countries and over time. The source is GLOBOCAN 2008, at http://globocan.iarc.fr.

Cancer registration is well established in a majority of European Union member states, although the quality and completeness of cancer registry data may vary. In some countries, cancer registries only cover subnational areas. The international comparability of cancer incidence data can also be affected by differences in medical training and practice.

The incidence of all cancers is classified to ICD-10 codes C00-C97, lung cancer to C33-C34, breast cancer to C50 and prostate cancer to C61.

1.13.1. All cancers incidence rates, males and females, 2008

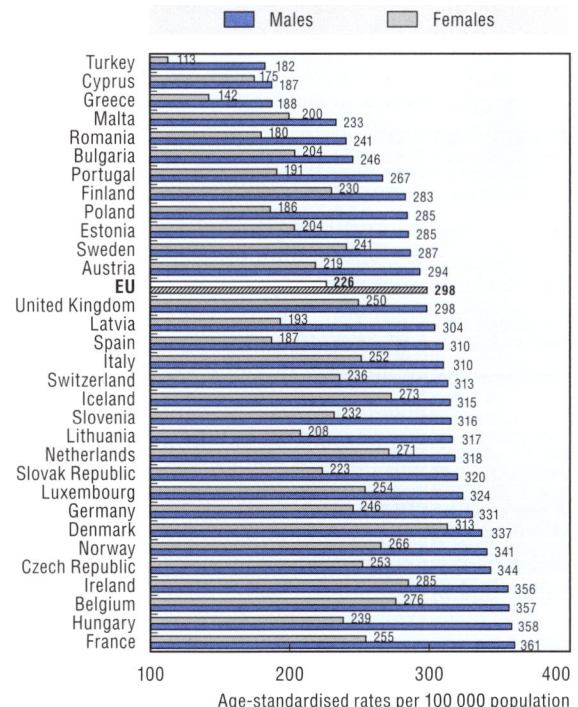

Age-standardised rates per 100 000 population

Source: OECD Health Data 2010; Ferlay et al. (2010).
StatLink ᵐˢᴾ http://dx.doi.org/10.1787/888932336046

1.13.2. Lung cancer incidence rates, males and females, 2008

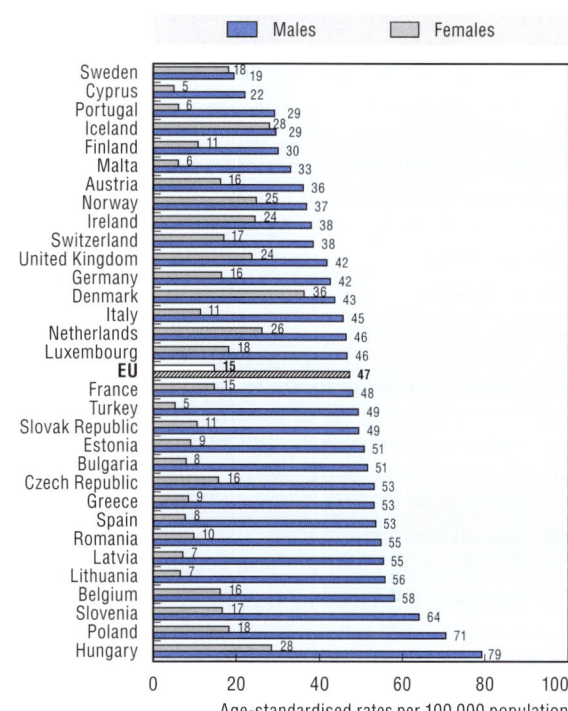

Age-standardised rates per 100 000 population

Source: OECD Health Data 2010; Ferlay et al. (2010).
StatLink ᵐˢᴾ http://dx.doi.org/10.1787/888932336065

1.13.3. Breast cancer incidence rates, females, 2008

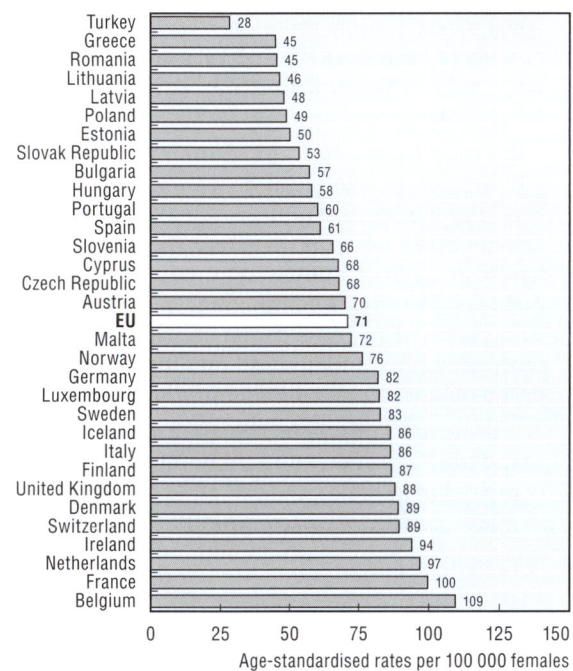

Age-standardised rates per 100 000 females

Source: OECD Health Data 2010; Ferlay et al. (2010).
StatLink ᵐˢᴾ http://dx.doi.org/10.1787/888932336084

1.13.4. Prostate cancer incidence rates, males, 2008

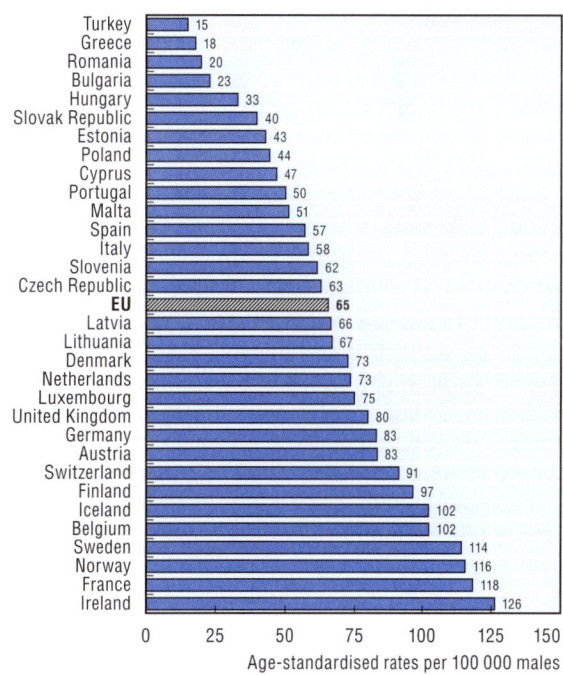

Age-standardised rates per 100 000 males

Source: OECD Health Data 2010; Ferlay et al. (2010).
StatLink ᵐˢᴾ http://dx.doi.org/10.1787/888932336103

Diabetes is a chronic metabolic disease, characterised by high levels of glucose in the blood. It occurs either because the pancreas stops producing the hormone insulin (type 1 diabetes), or through a combination of the pancreas having reduced ability to produce insulin alongside the body being resistant to its action (type 2 diabetes). People with diabetes are at a greater risk of developing cardiovascular diseases such as heart attack and stroke if the disease is left undiagnosed or poorly controlled. They also have elevated risks for sight loss, foot and leg amputation due to damage to the nerves and blood vessels, and renal failure requiring dialysis or transplantation.

Diabetes was the principal cause of death of more than 100 000 persons in EU countries in 2008, and is the fourth or fifth leading cause of death in most developed countries. However, only a minority of persons with diabetes die from diseases uniquely related to the condition – in addition, about 50% of persons with diabetes die of cardiovascular disease, and 10-20% of renal failure (IDF, 2006).

Diabetes is increasing rapidly in every part of the world, to the extent that it has now assumed epidemic proportions. Estimates suggest that more than 6% of the population aged 20-79 years in EU countries, or 33 million people, have diabetes in 2010. Almost half of diabetic adults are aged less than 60 years. If left unchecked, the number of people with diabetes in EU countries will reach more than 37 million in less than 20 years (IDF, 2006).

Less than 5% of adults aged 20-79 years in Iceland, Norway and the United Kingdom have diabetes, according to the International Diabetes Federation. This contrasts with Cyprus, Germany and Turkey, where 8% or more of the population of the same age have the disease (Figure 1.14.1). Among EU countries, abnormal glucose tolerance shows little association with affluence, and there was little evidence of an urban/rural divide in prevalence, except in a few countries (IDF, 2009).

Type 1 diabetes accounts for only 10-15% of all diabetes cases. It is the predominant form of the disease in younger age groups in most developed countries. Based on disease registers and recent studies, the annual number of new cases of type 1 diabetes in children aged under 15 years is high at 25 or more per 100 000 population in Nordic countries (Finland, Sweden and Norway) (Figure 1.14.2). Turkey,

Italy, Bulgaria and Greece have less than ten new cases per 100 000 population. Alarmingly, there is evidence that type 1 diabetes is developing at an earlier age among children.

The economic impact of diabetes is substantial. Health expenditure to treat and prevent diabetes and its complications is estimated to total USD 93 billion, or approximately 10% of total health expenditure in EU countries in 2010 (IDF, 2009). Around one-quarter of medical expenditure is spent on controlling elevated blood glucose, another quarter on treating long-term complication of diabetes, and the remainder on additional general medical care. Increasing costs reinforce the need to provide quality care for the management of diabetes and its complications.

Type 2 diabetes is largely preventable. A number of risk factors, such as overweight and obesity and physical inactivity are modifiable, and can also help reduce the complications that are associated with diabetes. But in most countries, the prevalence of overweight and obesity also continues to increase (see Indicator 2.8).

Definition and deviations

The sources and methods used by the International Diabetes Federation for publishing national prevalence estimates of diabetes are outlined in their *Diabetes Atlas*, 4th edition (IDF, 2009). Country data were derived from studies published between 1980 and February 2009, and were only included if they met several criteria for reliability.

Studies from several European countries – France, Italy, Netherlands, Norway, Slovenia and the United Kingdom – only provided self-reported data on diabetes. To account for undiagnosed diabetes, the prevalence of diabetes for the United Kingdom was multiplied by a factor of 1.5, in accordance with local recommendations, and doubled for other countries, based on data from a number of countries.

Prevalence rates were adjusted to the World Standard Population to facilitate cross-national comparisons.

1.14.1. Prevalence estimates of diabetes, adults aged 20-79 years, 2010

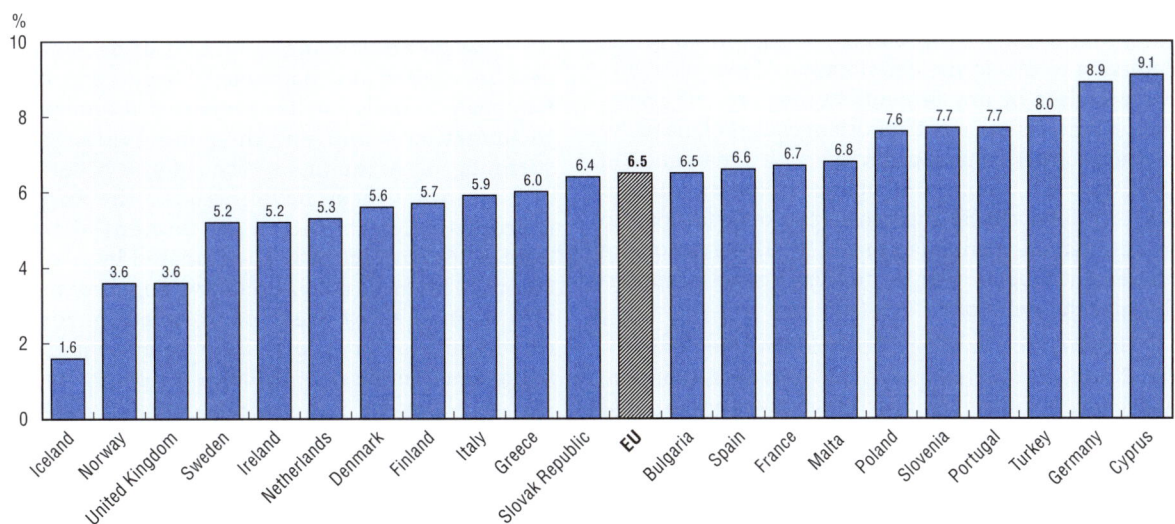

Note: The data are age-standardised to the World Standard Population.
Source: IDF (2009).

StatLink http://dx.doi.org/10.1787/888932336122

1.14.2. Incidence estimates of type 1 diabetes, children aged 0-14 years, 2010

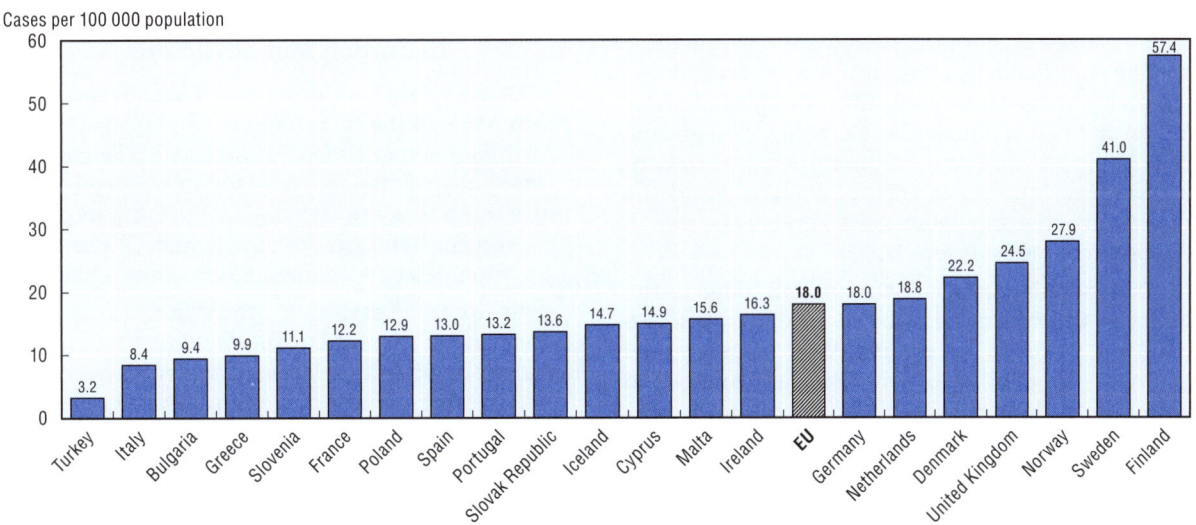

Source: IDF (2009).

StatLink http://dx.doi.org/10.1787/888932336141

Dementia describes a variety of brain disorders which progressively damage and destroy brain cells. Affecting mainly people over the age of 60 years, dementia results in the deterioration of mental ability characterised by impairments in memory and cognition. It is one of the most important causes of disability in the elderly. The most common cause of dementia in the European Union is Alzheimer's disease (around 50-70%), followed by successive strokes that lead to multi-infarct dementia (around 30%). There is no cure for dementia, but drugs exist to alleviate and temporarily delay the symptoms.

In 2006, the number of people with dementia in the European Union was estimated to be 7.3 million, and because of their longer life expectancy, almost 68% (4.9 million) of those affected were women. The highest prevalence rates were found in Sweden, Italy, Switzerland and Germany, where between 1.7-1.8% of the population suffer from dementia. This contrasts with less than 1.0% of the population in Turkey, the Slovak Republic and Ireland (Figure 1.15.1). The average dementia prevalence rate for the 27 EU countries was 1.4%.

Age is the main risk factor for the development of dementia. Although early-onset dementia can occur before the age of 65 years, prevalence rates increase steadily after that age, to reach 15% of males and 16% of females at age 80-84 years, and one-third of males (32.4%) and half of females (48.8%) at age 95 years and over (Figure 1.15.2). There is a strong positive relationship between the prevalence of dementia and the proportion of the population aged 65 years and over in European countries (Figure 1.15.3).

The population aged 65 years and older in the European Union is predicted to double between 1995 and 2050, to reach 135 million. With the increased ageing of the population, the absolute number of people with dementia will also continue to rise, placing greater demand on national health and social systems. Dementia places a large burden not only on sufferers, but also on their carers. Patterns of care vary across EU countries, with different mixes of informal care by families and friends, and formal care either in institutions or at home.

The cost of illness associated with Alzheimer's disease and other dementias in Europe was estimated at EUR 177 billion in 2006, which is divided fairly evenly between costs directly attributable to the diseases responsible for dementia, and estimates of costs associated with informal care. The total costs of dementia are expected to increase to over EUR 250 billion by 2030 (Alzheimer Europe, 2009).

One important cost driver is the increasing demand for institutional and residential care.

The prevention and treatment of dementia has been recognised as a major public health priority. The European Commission has supported several projects to investigate and enhance the evidence base surrounding Alzheimer's disease and other forms of dementia. These have included the EuroCoDe (European Collaboration on Dementia) project from 2006-08 which was co-ordinated by Alzheimer Europe. The most recent initiative supports national efforts in the key areas of prevention, research coordination and best practice in treatment and care (European Commission, 2010b).

At a national level, various countries including France, Norway and the United Kingdom have put in place national plans and strategies to meet the future challenges posed by dementia. These plans include measures to improve early diagnosis, treatment and the quality of care for people affected by dementia, as well as providing support to carers of those afflicted with dementia.

Definition and deviations

Dementia prevalence rates are based on estimates of the total number of persons living with dementia divided by the size of the corresponding population. The estimates of dementia prevalence were derived by the EuroCoDe (European Collaboration on Dementia) project, co-ordinated by Alzheimer Europe from 2006-08.

In order to estimate prevalence rates for dementia across European countries, the EuroCoDe project undertook a systematic review of papers reporting dementia prevalence estimates. Papers were screened according to criteria which stipulated that studies be community-based, use standardised diagnostic criteria, have a minimum sample size of 300 and a participation rate of over 50%, and be conducted in 1990 or thereafter. In addition, it was necessary that raw prevalence data be made available. Thirty-one studies met this criteria and raw data was extracted from 17 studies for use in the collaborative analysis.

Given the divergence in scale and accuracy of the sources used across countries, the prevalence estimates should be used with caution.

1.15.1. Prevalence of dementia, population aged 30 years and over, 2006

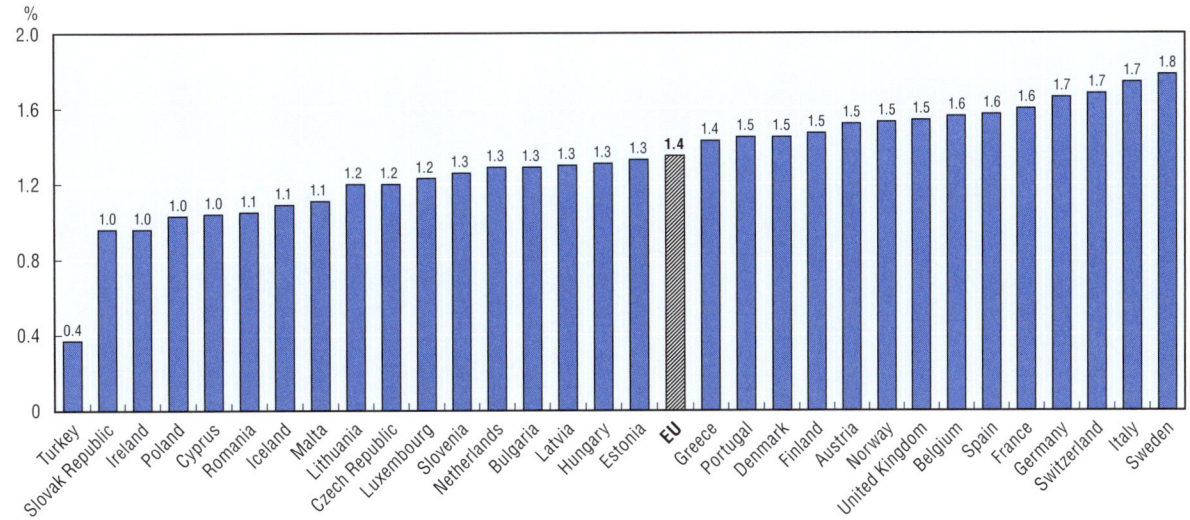

Source: Alzheimer Europe (2009).

StatLink ⟋⟍⟍ http://dx.doi.org/10.1787/888932336160

1.15.2. Age- and sex-specific prevalence of dementia in EU countries, 2006

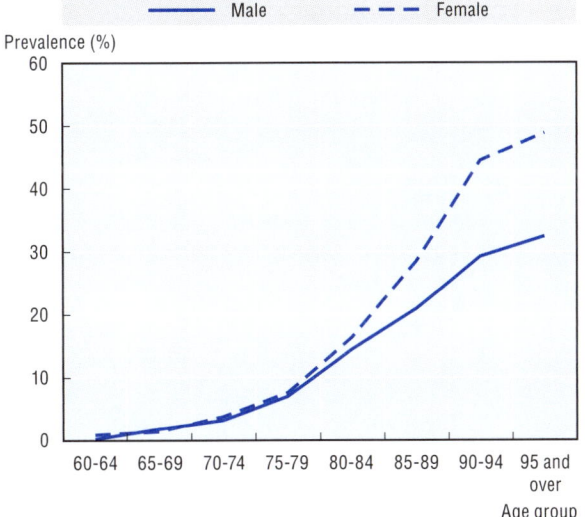

Source: Alzheimer Europe (2009).

StatLink ⟋⟍⟍ http://dx.doi.org/10.1787/888932336179

1.15.3. Population aged 65 years and over, and prevalence of dementia, 2006

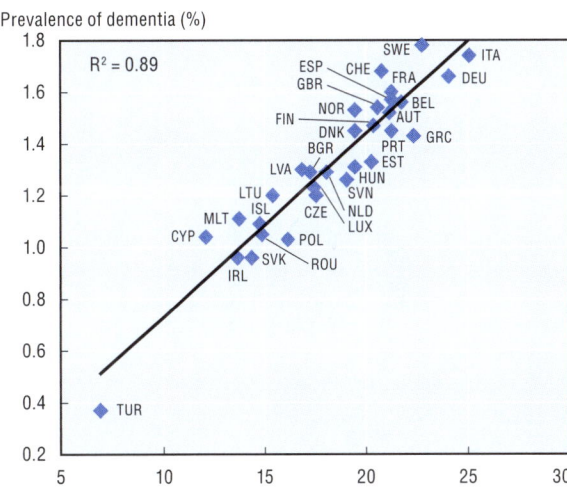

Source: Alzheimer Europe (2009); OECD Health Data 2010; Eurostat Statistics Database.

StatLink ⟋⟍⟍ http://dx.doi.org/10.1787/888932336198

Chapter 2

Determinants of Health

Regular smoking or excessive drinking in adolescence has both immediate and long-term health consequences. Children who establish smoking habits in early adolescence increase their risk of cardiovascular diseases, respiratory illnesses and cancer. They are also more likely to experiment with alcohol and other drugs. Alcohol misuse is itself associated with a range of social, physical and mental health problems, including depressive and anxiety disorders, obesity and accidental injury (Currie et al., 2008).

Results from the Health Behaviour in School-aged Children (HBSC) surveys, a series of collaborative cross-national studies conducted in most EU countries, allow for monitoring of smoking and drinking behaviours among adolescents. Generally, girls smoke more than boys, but more boys get drunk. Between 13 and 15 years of age, the prevalence of smoking and drunkenness doubles in many EU countries.

Boys and girls in central and eastern European countries (Bulgaria, Latvia, Estonia, Lithuania, the Czech Republic, Hungary) as well as in Austria, Finland and Italy smoke most often, with weekly rates around 20% or more (Figure 2.1.1). In contrast, 15% or less of 15-year-olds in Nordic countries (Denmark, Iceland, Norway and Sweden), Switzerland and Portugal smoke weekly. Many countries report higher rates of smoking for girls, although only Bulgaria, Austria and Spain have differences in excess of 5%. Smoking is more prevalent among boys in central and eastern European countries.

Drunkenness at least twice in their lifetime is reported by 40% or more of 15-year-olds in Denmark, Lithuania, the United Kingdom, Finland, Bulgaria and Estonia (Figure 2.1.2). Across all surveyed countries, 30% of girls and 38% of boys have been drunk on two or more occasions, with much lower rates in Mediterranean countries such as Malta, Greece, Portugal and Italy, as well as in Switzerland and France. Boys are more likely to report repeated drunkenness. Romania, Slovenia, Poland and Estonia have the biggest differences, with rates of alcohol abuse among boys being in excess of 15% higher than those of girls. Norway, Spain and the United Kingdom are the only countries where more girls report repeated drunkenness, and in each case rates are around 5% higher.

The differences in recent smoking and drinking rates between 15-year-old boys and girls are shown in Figure 2.1.3. Countries above the 45 degree line have higher rates for girls, and countries below the line higher rates for boys. Countries with higher rates of smoking among boys also report higher rates for girls, with the same finding for drinking rates.

Rates of drunkenness are also available for 13-year-olds (Currie et al., 2008). At this age, over one in ten children in a range of countries including Estonia, the United Kingdom, Lithuania, Latvia, Bulgaria, the Czech and Slovak Republics and Finland have experienced drunkenness at least twice. In Romania, Denmark and Slovenia, high rates of repeated drunkenness at 13 are also seen for boys. Some of the largest increases in reported drunkenness between the ages of 13 and 15 are seen in Denmark, Finland and Lithuania.

Risk-taking behaviours among adolescents are falling, with regular smoking for both boys and girls and drunkenness rates for boys showing some decline from the levels of the late 1990s (Figure 2.1.4). Levels of smoking for both sexes are at their lowest for a decade with, on average, fewer than one in five children of either sex smoking regularly. However, increasing rates of smoking and drunkenness among adolescents in Baltic and other eastern European countries are cause for concern.

Definition and deviations

Estimates for smoking refer to the proportion of 15-year-old children who self-report smoking at least once a week. Estimates for drunkenness record the proportions of 15-year-old children saying they have been drunk twice or more in their lives.

Data for 26 European Union and 3 non-EU countries are from the Health Behaviour in School-aged Children (HBSC) surveys undertaken between 1992-93 and 2005-06. Data are drawn from school-based samples. France, Germany and the United Kingdom report results for certain regions only. Turkey is included in the 2005-06 HBSC survey, but did not question children on drinking and smoking.

2.1.1. Smoking among 15-year-olds, 2005-06

Smoking at least once a week

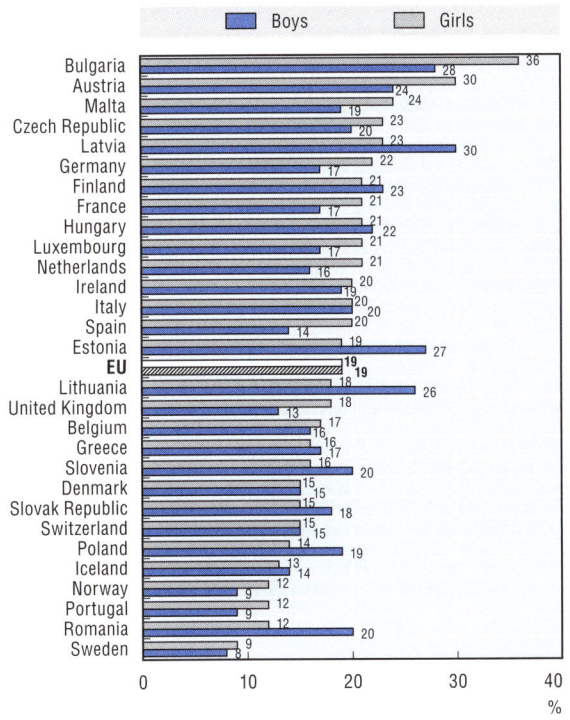

Source: Currie et al. (2008).

StatLink ⟹ http://dx.doi.org/10.1787/888932336217

2.1.2. Drunkenness among 15-year-olds, 2005-06

Drunk at least twice in life

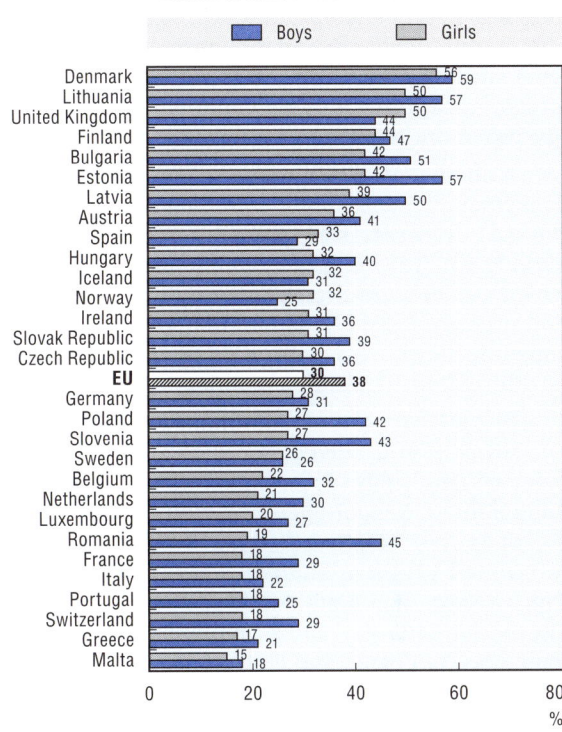

Source: Currie et al. (2008).

StatLink ⟹ http://dx.doi.org/10.1787/888932336236

2.1.3. Risk behaviours of 15-year-olds by sex, 2005-06

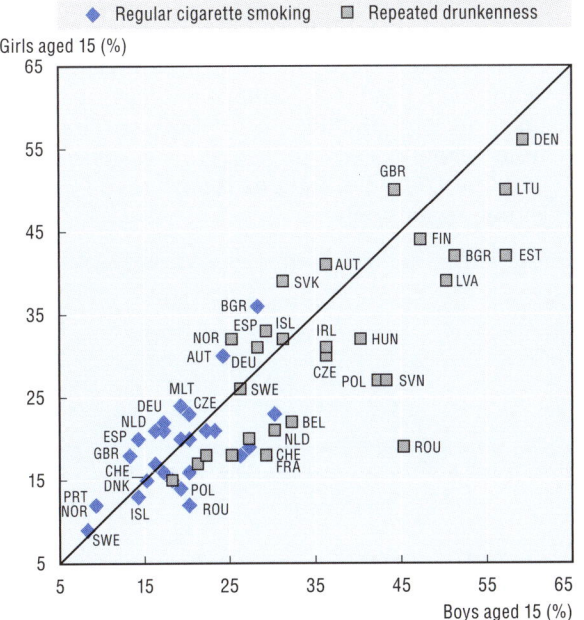

Source: Currie et al. (2008).

StatLink ⟹ http://dx.doi.org/10.1787/888932336255

2.1.4. Trends in repeated drunkenness and regular smoking among 15-year-olds, EU average

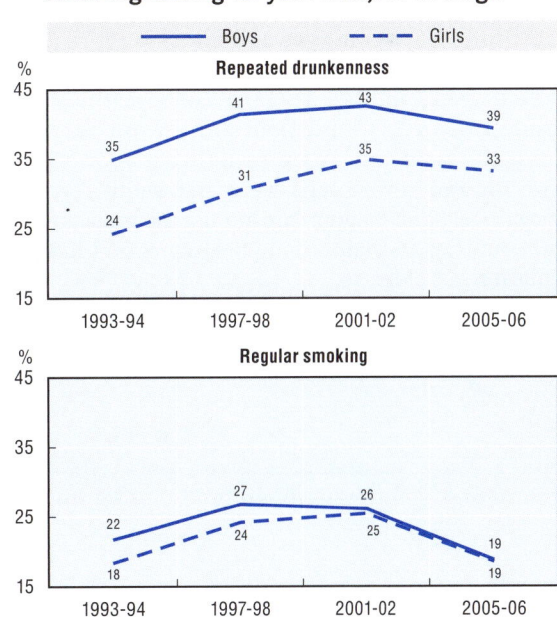

Source: Currie et al. (2000, 2004, 2008); WHO (1996).

StatLink ⟹ http://dx.doi.org/10.1787/888932336274

Nutrition is important for children's development and long-term health. Eating fruit during adolescence, for example, in place of high-fat, sugar and salt products, can protect against health problems such as obesity, diabetes, and heart problems. Moreover, eating fruit when young can be habit forming, promoting healthy eating behaviours for later life.

A number of factors influence the amount of fruit consumed by adolescents, including family income, the cost of alternatives, preparation time, whether parents eat fruit, and the availability of fresh fruit which can be linked to the country or local climate (Rasmussen *et al.*, 2006). Fruit (and vegetable) consumption have a high priority as indicators of healthy eating in most EU countries.

In 2005-06, only around one-third of boys and two-fifths of girls aged 11-15 years ate at least one piece of fruit daily, according to the latest Health Behaviour in School-aged Children (HBSC) survey (Currie *et al.*, 2008). Overall, boys in Italy, and girls in the United Kingdom had the highest rates of daily fruit consumption. Fruit consumption was relatively low among Baltic and some Nordic countries, including Latvia, Lithuania and Finland, with rates around one in four girls and one in five boys. At all ages and in most countries, girls were more likely to eat fruit daily. At age 11, girls in Norway, Portugal and Slovenia, as well as boys in Portugal, Italy and Bulgaria were more likely to eat fruit daily. By age 15, girls in Italy, Denmark and the United Kingdom, and boys in Italy, Portugal and Malta ate most (Figure 2.2.1).

In almost all EU countries, daily fruit consumption falls between ages 11 and 15 (Figure 2.2.2). Among girls, the EU average fell from 44% at age 11, to 39% at age 13 and 34% at age 15. For boys, the fall was from 37% to 32% and then 25%. In Bulgaria and Iceland, rates fell by up to half between ages 11 and 15, and severe falls were also seen in Austria (boys). Italy and Belgium are among the most successful countries in maintaining healthy eating habits as children get older.

The gap between the fruit consumption of boys and girls is largest at age 15, for most countries. At age 11, boys and girls in Lithuania as well as Italy, France and Estonia have similar rates of fruit consumption. Poland, Germany and the Netherlands have the biggest gaps at this age. As children reach age 15, gaps in Finland, Austria and Latvia grow to a level where fewer than six boys for every ten girls eat fruit regularly.

Average reported rates of daily fruit consumption across EU countries showed some increase between 2001-02 and 2005-06. This was most evident among girls aged 11 (Figure 2.2.3).

Effective strategies are required in order to ensure that children are eating enough fruit to conform with recommended dietary guidelines. Children generally hold a positive attitude toward fruit intake, and report good availability of fruit at home, but lower availability at school and during leisure time. Increased accessibility to fruit, combined with educational and motivational activities, can help in increasing fruit consumption (Sandvik *et al.*, 2005).

> ## Definition and deviations
>
> Nutrition is measured here in terms of the proportions of children who report eating fruit at least every day or more than once a day. In addition to fruit, healthy nutrition also involves other types of foods.
>
> Data for 26 European Union and four non-EU countries are from the Health Behaviour in School-aged Children (HBSC) surveys undertaken in 2001-02 and 2005-06. Data are drawn from school-based samples. France, Germany and the United Kingdom report results for certain regions only.

2.2.1. Daily fruit eating among 11- and 15-year-olds, 2005-06

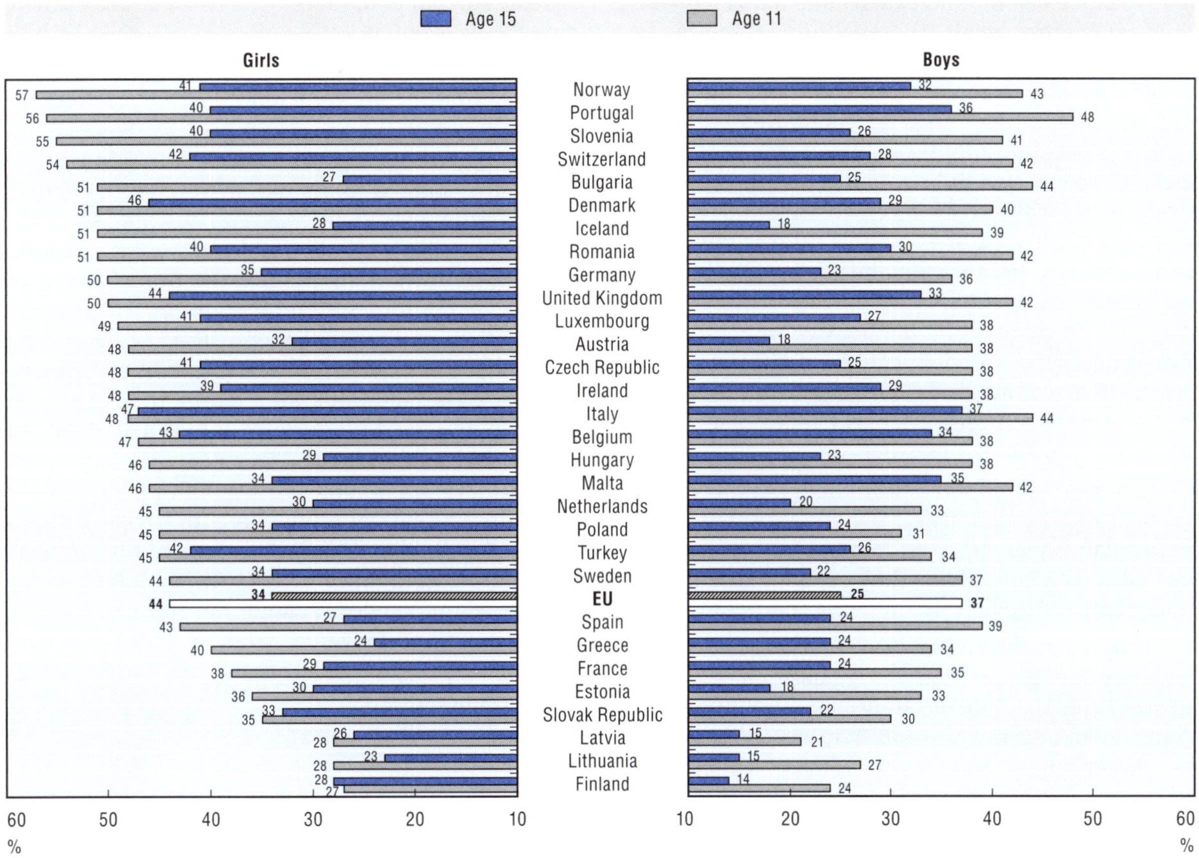

■ Age 15   □ Age 11

Girls

Country	Age 15	Age 11
Norway	41	57
Portugal	40	56
Slovenia	40	55
Switzerland	42	54
Bulgaria	27	51
Denmark	46	51
Iceland	28	51
Romania	40	51
Germany	35	50
United Kingdom	44	50
Luxembourg	41	49
Austria	32	48
Czech Republic	41	48
Ireland	39	48
Italy	47	48
Belgium	43	47
Hungary	29	46
Malta	34	46
Netherlands	30	45
Poland	34	45
Turkey	42	45
Sweden	34	44
EU	**34**	**44**
Spain	27	43
Greece	24	40
France	29	38
Estonia	30	36
Slovak Republic	33	35
Latvia	26	28
Lithuania	23	28
Finland	27	28

Boys

Country	Age 15	Age 11
Norway	32	43
Portugal	36	48
Slovenia	26	41
Switzerland	28	42
Bulgaria	25	44
Denmark	29	40
Iceland	18	39
Romania	30	42
Germany	23	36
United Kingdom	33	42
Luxembourg	27	38
Austria	18	38
Czech Republic	25	38
Ireland	29	38
Italy	37	44
Belgium	34	38
Hungary	23	38
Malta	35	42
Netherlands	20	33
Poland	24	31
Turkey	26	34
Sweden	22	37
EU	**25**	**37**
Spain	24	39
Greece	24	34
France	24	35
Estonia	18	33
Slovak Republic	22	30
Latvia	15	21
Lithuania	15	27
Finland	14	24

Source: Currie et al. (2008).

StatLink ᵐˢᵖ http://dx.doi.org/10.1787/888932336293

2.2.2. Regular fruit consumption at ages 11 and 15 years, 2005-06

◇ Girls   ■ Boys

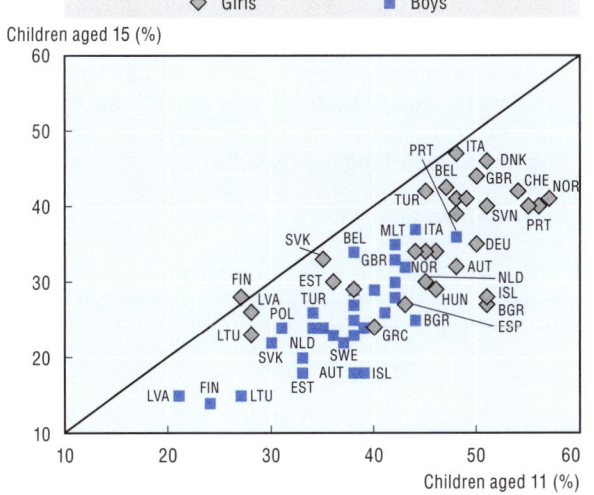

Source: Currie et al. (2008).
StatLink ᵐˢᵖ http://dx.doi.org/10.1787/888932336312

2.2.3. Average proportion of children in EU countries reporting daily fruit consumption, 2001-02 and 2005-06

■ Age 11   □ Age 13   ■ Age 15

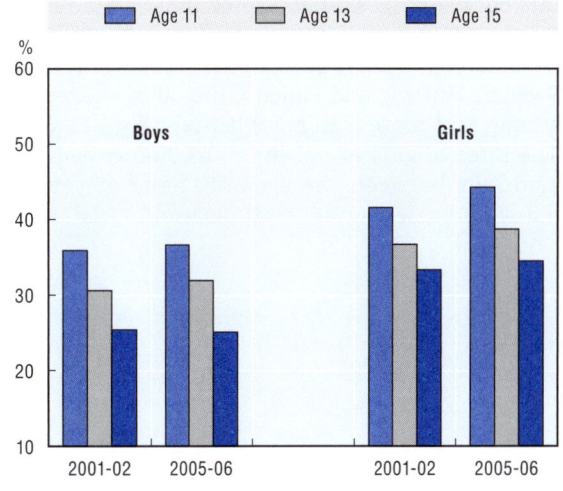

Source: Currie et al. (2004, 2008).
StatLink ᵐˢᵖ http://dx.doi.org/10.1787/888932336331

Undertaking physical activity in adolescence is beneficial for health, and can set standards for adult physical activity levels, thereby influencing health outcomes in later life. Research supports the role that physical activity in adolescence has in the prevention and treatment of a range of youth health issues including asthma, mental health, bone health and obesity. More direct links to adult health are found between physical activity in adolescence and its effect on overweight and obesity and related diseases, breast cancer rates and bone health in later life. The health effects of adolescent physical activity are sometimes dependent on the activity type, *e.g.* water physical activities in adolescence are effective in the treatment of asthma, and exercise is recommended in the treatment of cystic fibrosis (Hallal *et al.*, 2006; Currie *et al.*, 2008).

Some of the factors influencing the levels of physical activity undertaken by adolescents include the availability of space and equipment, the child's present health conditions, their school curricula and other competing pastimes.

Only one in five children in EU countries undertake moderate-to-vigorous exercise regularly, according to results from the 2005-06 HBSC survey. Children in Switzerland, Luxembourg and Italy are least likely to exercise regularly, whereas the Slovak Republic and Ireland stand out as strong performers with over 40 and 30% respectively of children aged 11 to 15 exercising for a total of at least 60 minutes per day over the past week (Figure 2.3.1). The country rankings reported vary according to the child's age. France appears at the lower end, especially for girls, at both ages. Boys consistently undertake more physical activity than girls, across all countries and all age groups.

It is of concern that physical activity tends to fall between ages 11 to 15 for most EU countries (Figure 2.3.2), with boys in the Czech Republic and Luxembourg the only exceptions. In Portugal, Norway, Sweden, Austria, and Finland, the rates of exercising among boys more than halve between ages 11 and 15. The rates of girls exercising to recommended levels also falls between the ages of 11 and 15 years. In many countries, rates for 15-year-old girls are less than half of those at age 11, and in Iceland, Romania, Ireland and Finland, rates of physical activity among girls fall by over 60%.

To compare levels of exercise between 2001-02 and 2005-06 for 15-year-old children, results are reported in relation to the EU average (Figure 2.3.3). In 2001-02, rates refer to 15-year-olds reporting an hour of moderate to vigorous exercise five days a week, but in 2005-06 figures refer to exercise of this type seven days a week. Boys' rates were above the EU average in the Netherlands, the United Kingdom, Greece, Spain and Switzerland in 2001-02, but fell below the average in 2005-06. Latvia, Belgium and Denmark are countries where rates of physical activity were below the EU average in 2001-02, but were among the higher performers in 2005-06. For 15-year-old boys, only the Czech Republic, Ireland and Poland have been consistently high performers on measures of physical activity in both waves. For girls, Latvia, Belgium and Malta have moved from below average performances in 2001-02 to above average in 2005-06. In Sweden, Poland, the United Kingdom, Switzerland and Slovenia, rates of physical activity among 15-year-old girls have fallen below the EU average since 2001-02.

Definition and deviations

Data for physical activity considers the regularity of moderate-to-vigorous physical activity as reported by 11- and 15-year-olds for the years 2001-02 and 2005-06. Moderate-to-vigorous physical activity refers to exercise undertaken for at least an hour which increases both heart rate and respiration (and leaves the child out of breath sometimes) on five or more days per week in 2001-02, and seven days a week in 2005-06.

Indicators are taken from the Health Behaviour in School-aged Children Survey (HBSC). Data are drawn from school-based samples, but some countries report regional results only.

2.3.1. Children aged 11 and 15 years doing moderate-to-vigorous physical activity daily in the past week, 2005-06

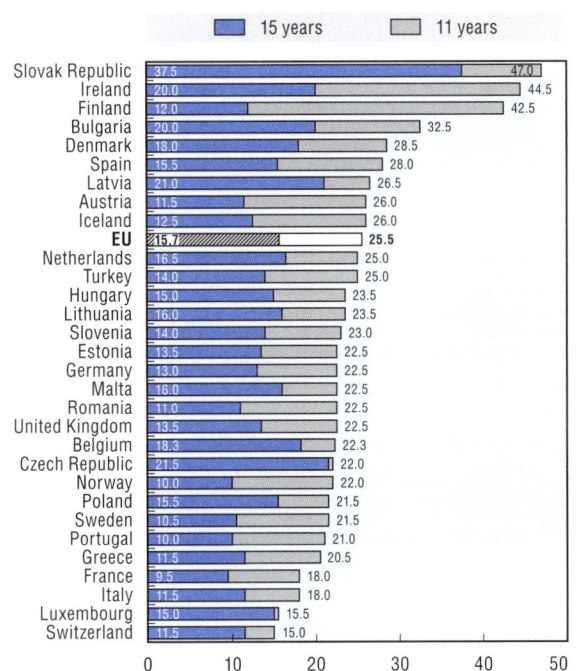

Source: Currie et al. (2008).

StatLink http://dx.doi.org/10.1787/888932336350

2.3.2. Comparing physical activity of 11- and 15-year-old children by sex, 2005-06

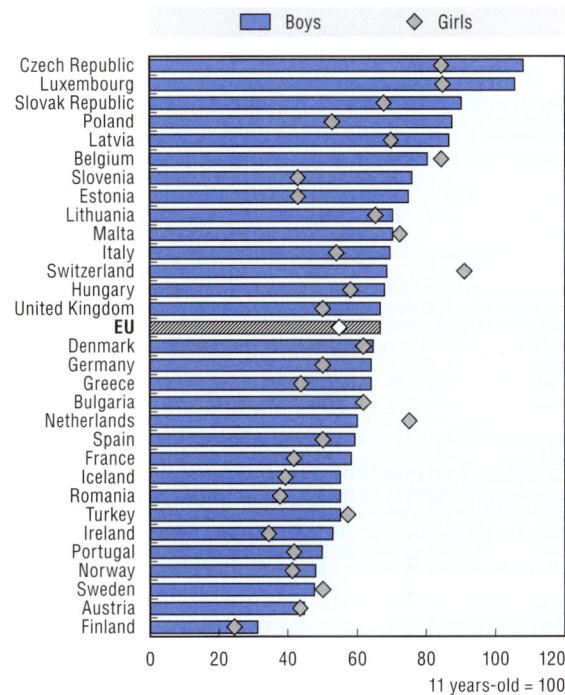

Source: Currie et al. (2008).

StatLink http://dx.doi.org/10.1787/888932336369

2.3.3. Standardised rates of physical activity for 15-year-old children (EU average = 1), 2001-02 and 2005-06

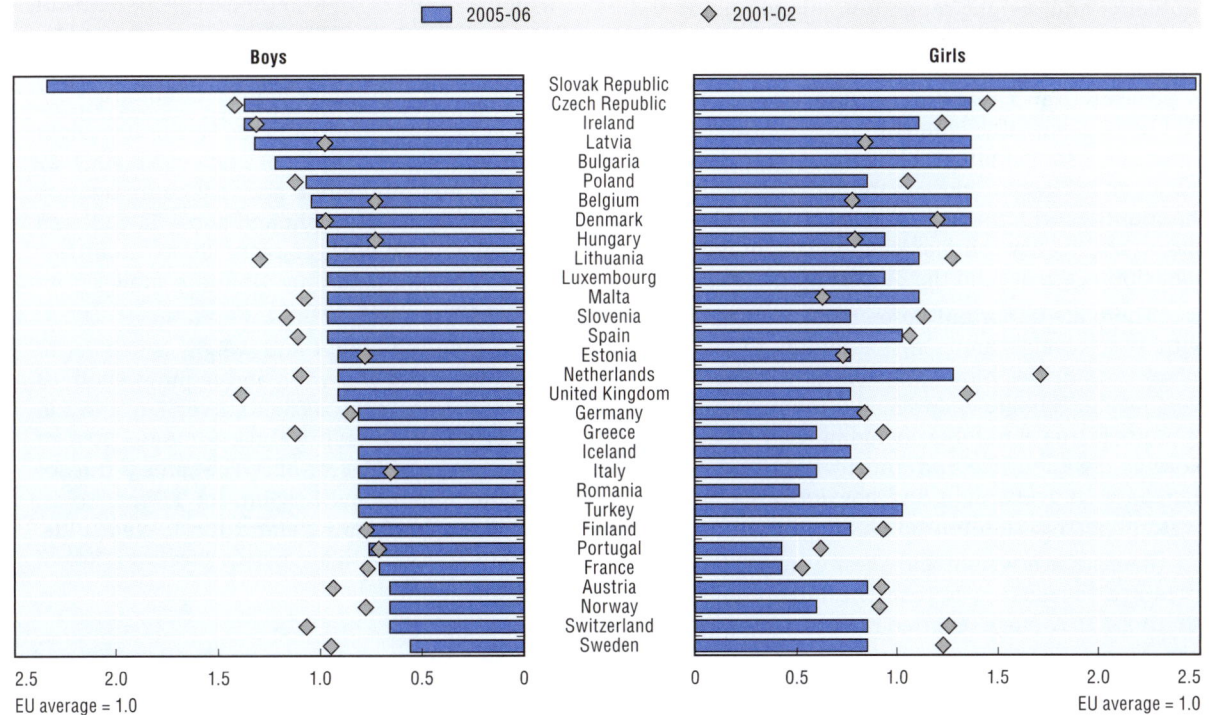

Source: Currie et al. (2004, 2008).

StatLink http://dx.doi.org/10.1787/888932336388

Children who are overweight or obese are at greater risk of poor health in adolescence and also in adulthood. Being overweight in childhood increases the risk of developing cardiovascular disease or diabetes, as well as related social and mental health problems. Excess weight problems in childhood are associated with an increased risk of being an obese adult, at which point certain forms of cancer, osteoarthritis, a reduced quality of life and premature death can be added to the list of health concerns (OECD, 2010c; Currie et al., 2008).

Evidence suggests that even if excess childhood weight is lost, adults who were obese children retain an increased risk of cardiovascular problems. And although dieting can combat obesity, children who diet are at a greater risk of putting on weight following periods of dieting. Eating disorders, symptoms of stress and postponed physical development can also be products of dieting.

Across most EU countries, one in seven children are overweight or obese (Figure 2.4.1). Aggregate figures for 2005-06 show that nearly one in five children in southern European countries (Malta, Greece, Portugal, Italy and Spain), are overweight or obese. Fewer than one in ten children in selected eastern European countries (Lithuania, Latvia, the Slovak Republic and Estonia) as well as in the Netherlands, Switzerland and Denmark are overweight or obese.

There is no clear association between weight problems and weight reduction behaviours at the national level. In most countries, the number of children who say that they are trying to lose weight is greater than the number with excess weight problems. Generally, countries where few children report excess weight problems also report weight reduction behaviours close to the EU average. Many of the countries with the highest rates of overweight and obese children have similar levels of weight reduction behaviour, each around the EU average of 13%.

There are important differences among children with excess weight problems, according to their age. In some countries older children have more excess weight than younger children, for other countries the opposite is true. A number, including the Netherlands, Norway, Sweden, Iceland and Switzerland, report increases in overweight and obesity rates for both boys and girls as children get older.

Rates of overweight and obesity among boys and girls are increasing across the European Union (Chart 2.4.2). Average reported rates of overweight and obesity increased between 2001-02 and 2005-06 from 12% to 16% for 15-year-old boys, and from 7% to 9% for girls. Between 2001-02 and 2005-06, every surveyed country reported an increase in overweight or obesity for boys aged 15. The largest increases during the four year period were found in Austria, Lithuania and Poland. A similar pattern of increases is seen for girls, with rates in Portugal and Germany almost doubling. Only Ireland, Norway and the United Kingdom report reductions in the proportion of overweight or obese girls at age 15 between 2001-02 and 2005-06. However, because non-response rates to questions of self-reported height and weight were high in these countries, cautious interpretation is required.

Childhood is an important period for forming healthy behaviours. Schools provide an opportunity to ensure that children understand the importance of good nutrition and physical activity, and can benefit from both. Studies show that locally focussed actions and interventions, targeting 0-12 year-olds can be effective in changing behaviours.

Definition and deviations

Estimates of overweight and obesity are based on Body Mass Index (BMI) calculations using child self-reported height and weight. Overweight and obese children are those whose BMI is above a set of age- and sex-specific cut-off points (Cole et al., 2000). Data on weight reduction record children who report being on a diet or doing something else to lose weight.

Indicators are taken from the Health Behaviour in School-aged Children Surveys in 2001-02 and 2005-06. Aggregate country estimates are crude rates of overweight and obese 11-, 13- and 15-year-olds in each country. Some countries report regional data only. Data are drawn from school-based samples.

Self-reported height and weight is subject to under-reporting and error, and requires cautious interpretation. In the 2005-06 survey, England and Norway have missing data for over 30% of respondents for 11-year-olds. The same is true for England, Ireland and Belgium for 13-years-olds, and in England and Ireland for 15-year-olds. In 2001-02, BMI data are missing for over 30% of respondents in Ireland.

2.4.1. Children aged 11-15 years who are overweight or obese, and children who are involved in weight-reduction behaviour, 2005-06

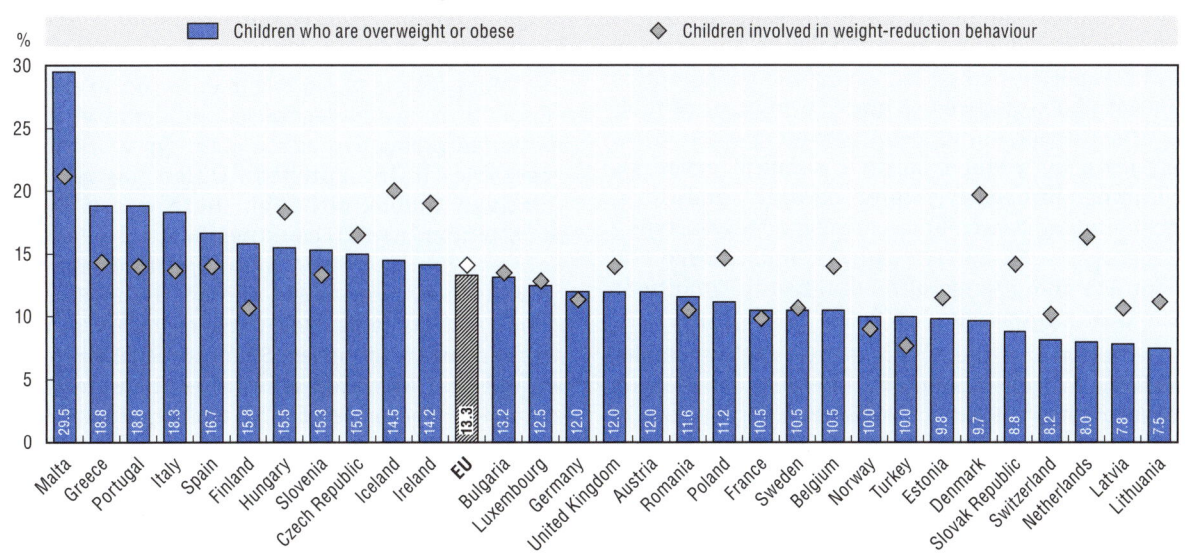

Children who are overweight or obese
Children involved in weight-reduction behaviour
%
30
25
20
15
10
5
0
29.5
18.8
18.8
18.3
16.7
15.8
15.5
15.3
15.0
14.5
14.2
13.3
13.2
12.5
12.0
12.0
12.0
11.6
11.2
10.5
10.5
10.5
10.0
10.0
9.8
9.7
8.8
8.2
8.0
7.8
7.5
Malta
Greece
Portugal
Italy
Spain
Finland
Hungary
Slovenia
Czech Republic
Iceland
Ireland
EU
Bulgaria
Luxembourg
Germany
United Kingdom
Austria
Romania
Poland
France
Sweden
Belgium
Norway
Turkey
Estonia
Denmark
Slovak Republic
Switzerland
Netherlands
Latvia
Lithuania

Source: Currie *et al.* (2004, 2008).

StatLink http://dx.doi.org/10.1787/888932336407

2.4.2. Change in obesity rates between 2001-02 and 2005-06, for 15-year-old boys and girls

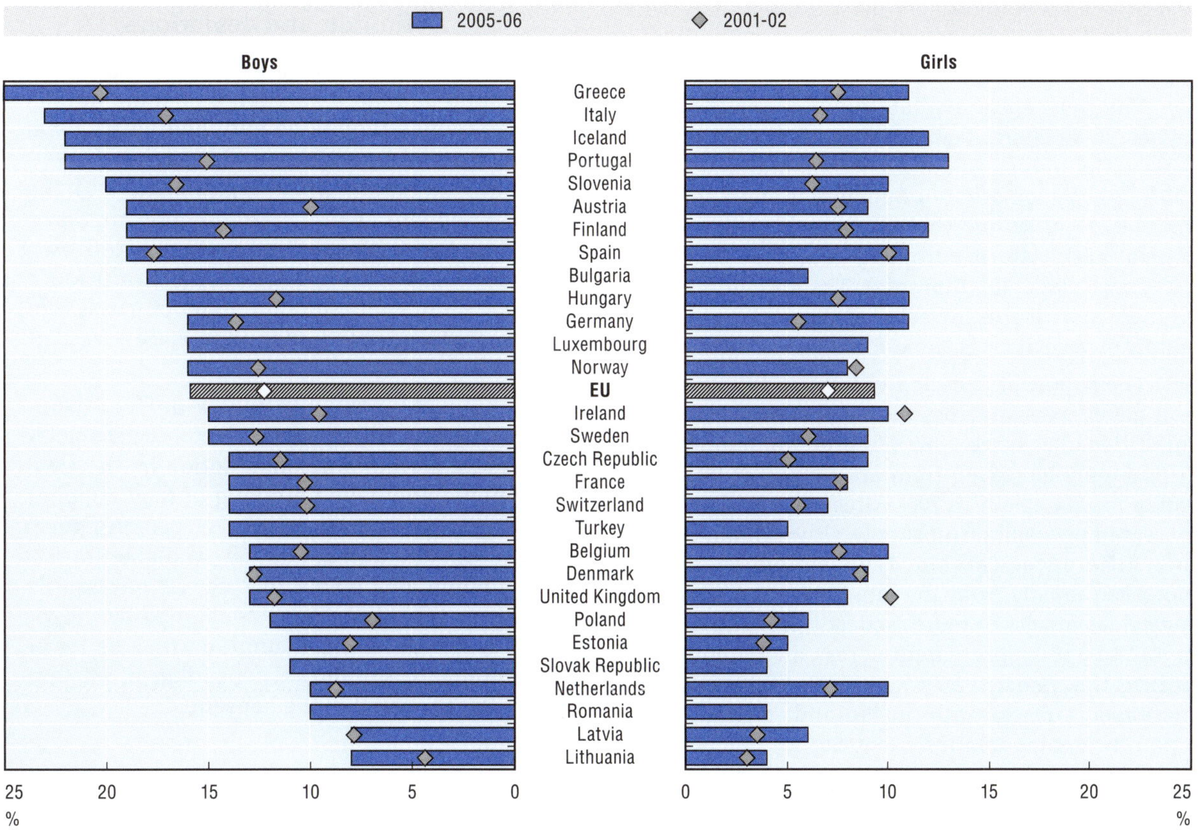

2005-06
2001-02
Boys
Girls
Greece
Italy
Iceland
Portugal
Slovenia
Austria
Finland
Spain
Bulgaria
Hungary
Germany
Luxembourg
Norway
EU
Ireland
Sweden
Czech Republic
France
Switzerland
Turkey
Belgium
Denmark
United Kingdom
Poland
Estonia
Slovak Republic
Netherlands
Romania
Latvia
Lithuania
25
20
15
10
5
0
%
0
5
10
15
20
25
%

Source: Currie *et al.* (2004, 2008).

StatLink http://dx.doi.org/10.1787/888932336426

Nutrition is an important determinant of health. Inadequate consumption of fruit and vegetables is one factor that can play a role in increased morbidity and premature death. A recent European Commission White Paper advocated increasing the consumption of fruit and vegetables as one of a number of tools to offset a worsening trend of poor diets and low physical activity. Proper nutrition assists in preventing a number of obesity-related chronic conditions, including cardiovascular disease, hypertension, type 2 diabetes, stroke, certain cancers, musculoskeletal disorders and a range of mental health conditions (European Commission, 2007).

Estimates of the supply of fruit and vegetables available for consumption in different countries are calculated by the Food and Agriculture Organization of the United Nations (FAO). In 2007, levels of the supply of both fruit and vegetables differed substantially across European countries (Figure 2.5.1). The per capita fruit supply in a number of central and eastern European countries, including Poland, Bulgaria, Romania, Latvia, the Slovak Republic, the Czech Republic and Estonia, was below 80 kg per person, contrasting with an EU average of 105. Fruit supply was greater in Western and Southern Europe, with estimates for Luxembourg and Greece above 160 kg per person, more than twice the amount of those countries reporting the lowest supply.

The per capita availability of vegetables was highest in Mediterranean countries, including Greece, Turkey, Malta, Portugal, Spain, Italy and Cyprus, all at 150 kg per person or more. Supply was lower than the EU average in Nordic countries, as well as in some central and eastern European countries (Bulgaria, the Czech Republic, Slovenia). The spread between countries with the lowest and highest per capita supply of vegetables is three-fold.

The supply of fruit and vegetables for consumption has increased across the European Union in the three decades since 1980 (Figures 2.5.2 and 2.5.3). Fruit supply increased from an average of 88 kg per capita in 1980 to 105 in 2007. Greece and Poland both increased per capita fruit supply, although large absolute differences remain. Fruit supply in Ireland increased rapidly from the late 1990s. The supply of vegetables increased more modestly, from an average of 102 to 116 kg per capita across all EU countries during the years 1980 to 2007. Vegetable supply increased substantially in Finland, although the amount remains relatively low. Supply has changed

little in Greece, but levels per capita vegetable remain the highest. In contrast, the supply of vegetables in Bulgaria has declined recently to one of the lowest levels among member states.

Many factors play a role in ensuring an adequate supply of fruit and vegetables. In recent years, the harvested production of the main types of fruit and vegetables in the European Union has remained relatively stable, although there was growth in imports from non-EU countries (Martinez-Palou and Rohner-Thielen, 2008). The majority of suppliers growing fresh vegetables are located in Romania, Poland and Lithuania. Most citrus farms are located in Mediterranean countries (Spain, Greece, Italy), with Poland and Romania also large fruit-producing countries. The price of fruit and vegetables varies considerably among member states. In 2006, for example, it was almost half the EU average in Bulgaria and a number of other eastern European countries adjusted by purchasing power parity, but more than 20% higher in Ireland, Luxembourg and Nordic countries (Denmark, Finland, Sweden) (Martinez-Palou and Rohner-Thielen, 2008).

Definition and deviations

Estimates of food available for consumption are based on annual production and trade of food commodities figures as supplied by national Ministries of Agriculture and Trade to the FAO (Food and Agriculture Organization of the United Nations). Gross apparent consumption = (Commercial production + estimated own account production for self-consumption + imports + opening stocks) – (exports + usage for processed food + feed + non-food usage + wastage + closing stocks).

Per person consumption is derived from dividing the total amount of fruit and vegetables available for human consumption by the total population actually partaking of food supplies during the reference period. Per person figures represent the average supply available for the population as a whole, and do not necessarily indicate what is actually consumed by individuals. Actual food consumption may be lower than the quantity shown, depending on wastage and losses of food in the household.

2.5.1. Supply of fruit and vegetables for consumption, 2007

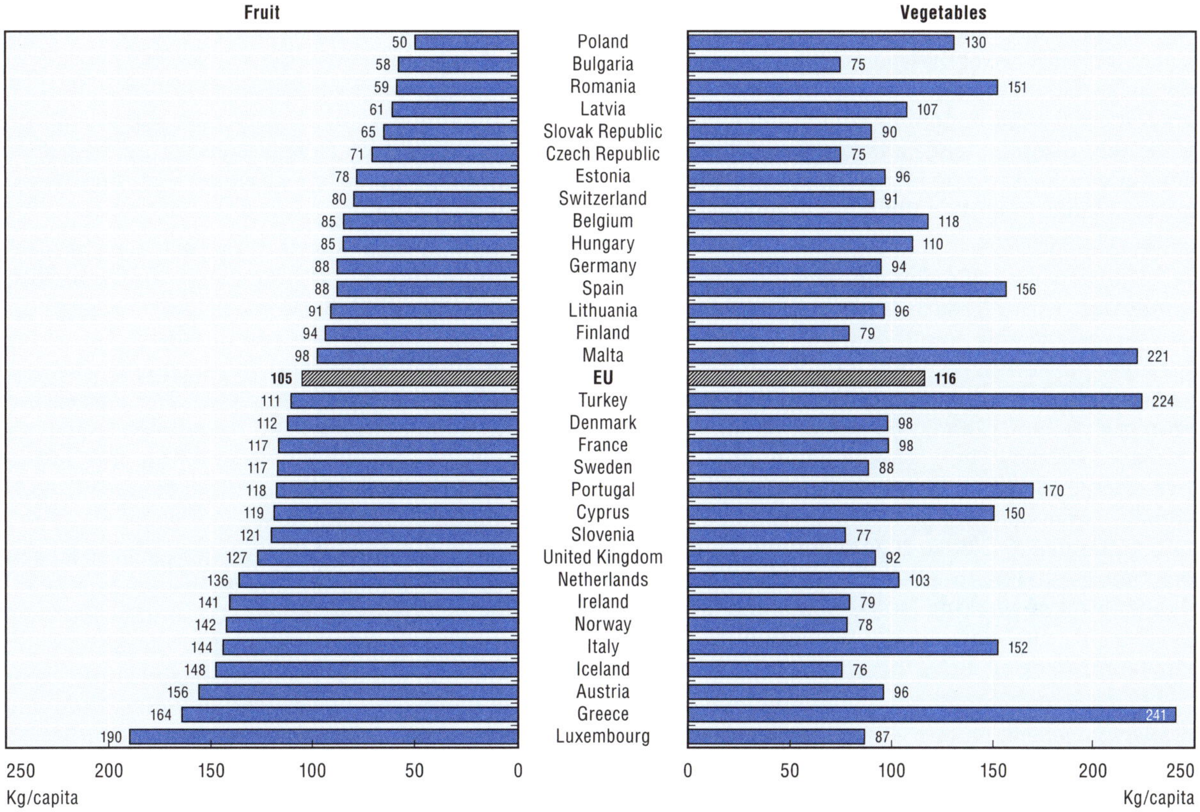

Fruit
Vegetables
Poland 50 130
Bulgaria 58 75
Romania 59 151
Latvia 61 107
Slovak Republic 65 90
Czech Republic 71 75
Estonia 78 96
Switzerland 80 91
Belgium 85 118
Hungary 85 110
Germany 88 94
Spain 88 156
Lithuania 91 96
Finland 94 79
Malta 98 221
EU 105 116
Turkey 111 224
Denmark 112 98
France 117 98
Sweden 117 88
Portugal 118 170
Cyprus 119 150
Slovenia 121 77
United Kingdom 127 92
Netherlands 136 103
Ireland 141 79
Norway 142 78
Italy 144 152
Iceland 148 76
Austria 156 96
Greece 164 241
Luxembourg 190 87
250
200
150
100
50
0
Kg/capita

Source: *FAOSTAT Database; OECD Health Data 2010.*

StatLink http://dx.doi.org/10.1787/888932336445

2.5.2. Trends in supply of fruit, selected EU countries, 1980-2007

Greece
Ireland
Poland
EU
Kg/capita/year
200
150
100
50
0
1980
1985
1990
1995
2000
2005

Source: *FAOSTAT Database; OECD Health Data 2010.*

StatLink http://dx.doi.org/10.1787/888932336464

2.5.3. Trends in supply of vegetables, selected EU countries, 1980-2007

Bulgaria
Greece
Finland
EU
Kg/capita/year
400
300
200
100
0
1980
1985
1990
1995
2000
2005

Source: *FAOSTAT Database; OECD Health Data 2010.*

StatLink http://dx.doi.org/10.1787/888932336483

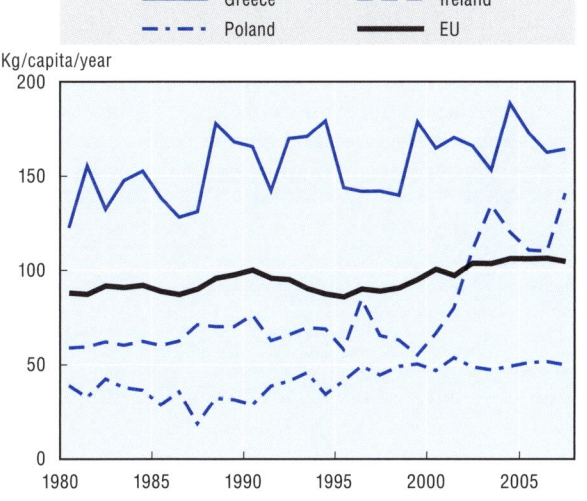

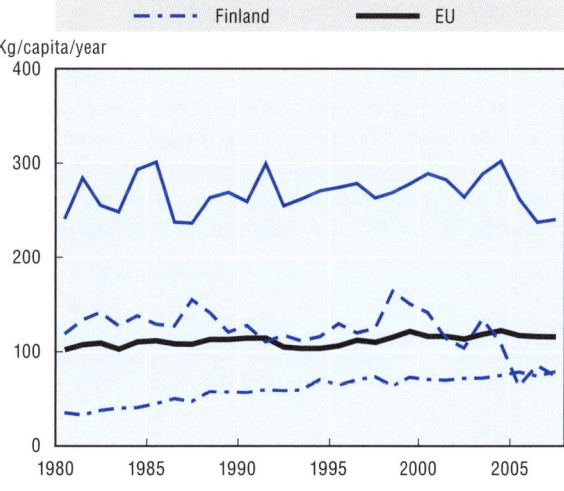

Tobacco is directly responsible for about one in ten adult deaths worldwide, equating to about 6 million deaths each year (Shafey *et al.*, 2009). It is a major risk factor for at least two of the leading causes of premature mortality – circulatory diseases and a range of cancers. In addition, it is an important contributory factor for respiratory diseases, while smoking among pregnant women can lead to low birth weight and illnesses among infants. It remains the largest avoidable risk to health in EU countries.

The proportion of daily smokers among the adult population varies greatly across countries, even between neighboring countries (Figure 2.6.1). In 2008, rates were lowest in Sweden, Iceland, Slovenia and Portugal, all at less than 20% of the adult population smoking daily. On average, smoking rates have decreased by about 5 percentage points in EU countries since 1995, with a bigger decline in men than in women. Large declines occurred in Turkey (47% to 27%), Luxembourg (33% to 20%), Norway (33% to 21%) and Denmark (36% to 23%). Greece maintains the highest level of smoking (40%), along with Bulgaria and Ireland, with close to 30% or more of the adult population smoking daily.

In the post-war period, most EU countries tended to follow a general pattern – very high smoking rates among men (50% or more) through to the 1960s and 1970s, while the 1980s and the 1990s were characterised by a marked downturn in tobacco consumption. Much of this decline can be attributed to policies aimed at reducing tobacco consumption through public awareness campaigns, advertising bans and increased taxation (World Bank, 1999). In addition to government policies, actions by anti-smoking interest groups were very effective in reducing smoking rates by changing beliefs about the health effects of smoking.

Although large disparities remain, this pattern of a decline in smoking rates is found across most EU countries (Figure 2.6.2). Smoking prevalence among men continues to be higher than among women in all EU countries except Sweden. Female smoking rates continue to decline in most countries, and in a number of cases (Turkey, Iceland, Belgium, Latvia and Ireland)

at an even faster pace than male rates. However, in seven countries, female smoking rates have been increasing since the mid-1990s (Lithuania, Portugal, Greece, Bulgaria, France, Germany and Austria), but even in these countries women are still less likely to smoke than men. In 2008, the gender gap in smoking rates was particularly large in Baltic countries (Latvia, Lithuania and Estonia), as well as in Turkey and Romania (Figure 2.6.1).

Several studies provide strong evidence of socio-economic differences in smoking and mortality (Mackenbach *et al.*, 2008). People in lower social groups have a greater prevalence and intensity of smoking, a higher all-cause mortality rate and lower rates of cancer survival (Woods *et al.*, 2006). The influence of smoking as a determinant of overall health inequalities is such that, in a non-smoking population, mortality differences between social groups would be halved (Jha *et al.*, 2006).

Figure 2.6.3 shows the correlation between tobacco consumption (as measured by grams per capita) and incidence of lung cancer across EU countries for which data are available, with a time lag of two decades. Higher tobacco consumption at the national level is also generally associated with higher mortality rates from lung cancer one or two decades later across EU countries.

Definition and deviations

The proportion of daily smokers is defined as the percentage of the population aged 15 years and over reporting smoking every day.

International comparability is limited due to the lack of standardisation in the measurement of smoking habits in health interview surveys across EU countries. Variations remain in the age groups surveyed, wording of questions, response categories and survey methodologies, *e.g.* in a number of countries, respondents are asked if they smoke regularly, rather than daily.

2.6.1. Daily smoking rates, 2008 (or nearest year available)

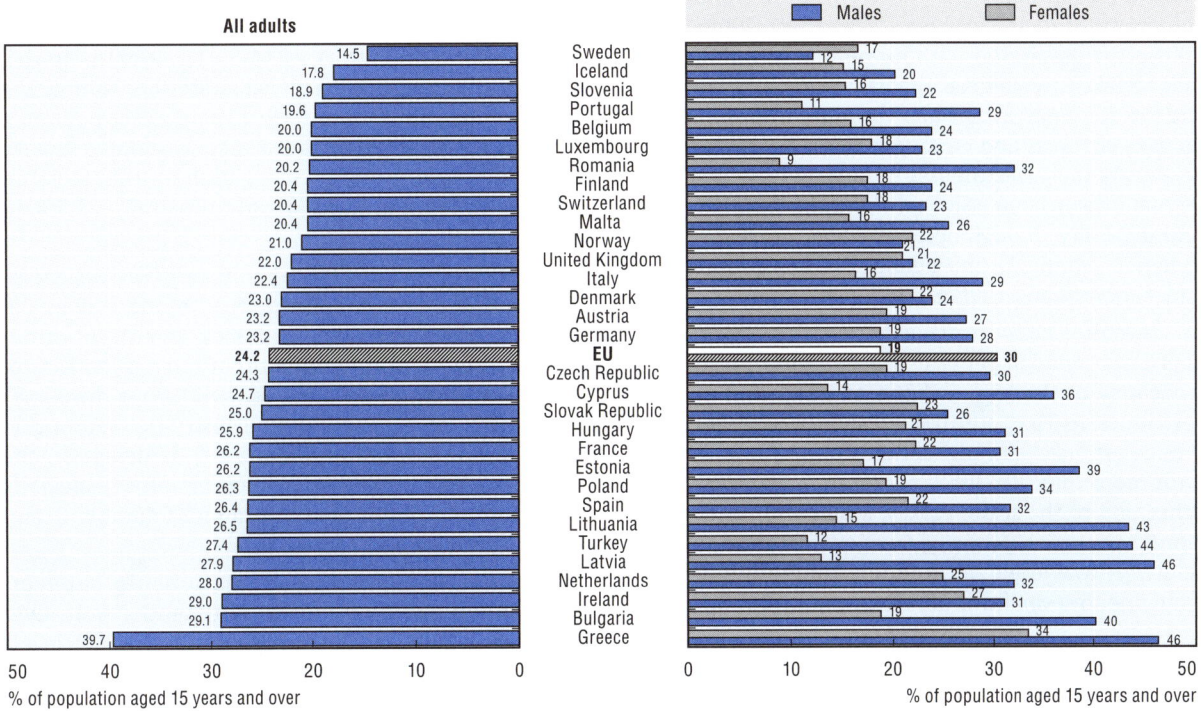

Source: OECD Health Data 2010; Eurostat Statistics Database.

StatLink http://dx.doi.org/10.1787/888932336502

2.6.2. Change in smoking rates by gender, 1995-2008 (or nearest year available)

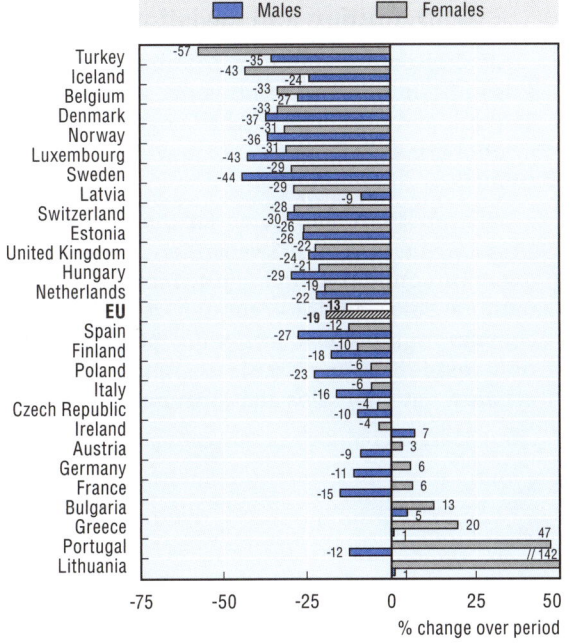

Source: OECD Health Data 2010; Eurostat Statistics Database; WHO Global Infobase.

StatLink http://dx.doi.org/10.1787/888932336521

2.6.3. Tobacco consumption, 1990 and incidence of lung cancer, 2008

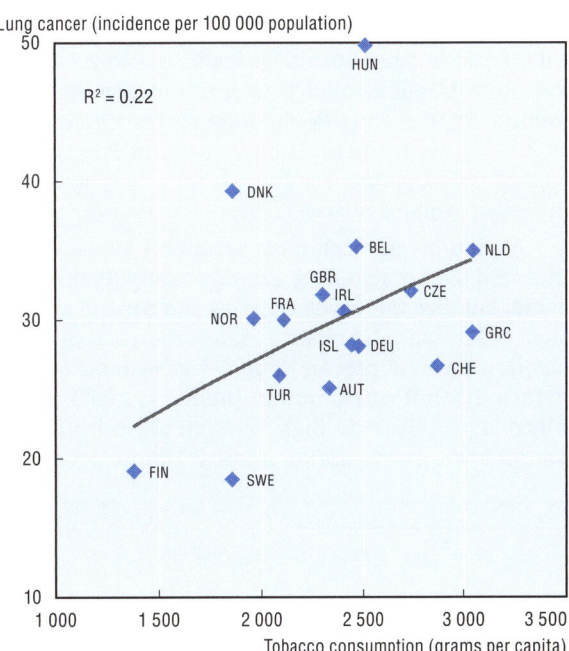

Source: OECD Health Data 2010.

StatLink http://dx.doi.org/10.1787/888932336540

The global health burden related to excessive alcohol consumption, both in terms of morbidity and mortality, is considerable (Rehm *et al.*, 2009; WHO, 2004). It is associated with numerous harmful health and social consequences. High alcohol intake increases the risk for heart, stroke and vascular diseases, as well as liver cirrhosis and certain cancers. Foetal exposure to alcohol increases the risk of birth defects and intellectual impairments. Alcohol also contributes to death and disability through accidents and injuries, assault, violence, homicide and suicide, and is estimated to cause more than 2 million deaths annually.

Alcohol consumption across EU countries is 10.8 litres per adult per year. Leaving aside Luxembourg – because of the high volume of purchases by non-residents in that country – Estonia, Hungary and France reported the highest consumption of alcohol, with more than 12.5 litres per adult in 2007-08. At the other end of the scale, Turkey, Malta and some of the Nordic countries (Norway, Sweden and Iceland) have relatively low levels of alcohol consumption, ranging from one to seven litres per adult (Figure 2.7.1).

Although average alcohol consumption has gradually fallen in many EU countries over the past three decades, it has risen in some others (Figure 2.7.1). There has been a degree of convergence in drinking habits across the European Union, with wine consumption increasing in many traditional beer-drinking countries and *vice versa*. The traditional wine-producing countries of Italy, France and Spain, as well as the Slovak Republic, Greece and Germany have seen their alcohol consumption per capita fall substantially since 1980 (Figures 2.7.1 and 2.7.2). On the other hand, alcohol consumption per capita in Iceland, Cyprus, Finland and Ireland rose by as much as 30% or more since 1980 although, in the case of Iceland and Cyprus, it started from a low level and therefore remains relatively low.

Variations in alcohol consumption across countries and over time reflect not only changing drinking habits but also the policy responses to control alcohol use. Curbs on advertising, sales restrictions and taxation have all proven to be effective measures to reduce alcohol consumption (Bennett, 2003). Strict controls on sales and high taxation are mirrored by overall lower consumption in most Nordic countries,

while falls in consumption in France, Italy and Spain may be associated with the voluntary and statutory regulation of advertising, partly following a 1989 European directive. In 2010, the World Health Organization endorsed a global strategy to combat the harmful use of alcohol, through direct measures such as medical services for alcohol-related health problems, and indirect ones, such as the dissemination of information on alcohol-related harm (WHO, 2010c).

Although adult alcohol consumption per capita gives useful evidence of long-term trends, it does not identify sub-populations at risk from harmful drinking patterns. The consumption of large quantities of alcohol at a single session, termed "binge drinking", is a particularly dangerous pattern of consumption (Institute of Alcohol Studies, 2007), which is on the rise in some countries and social groups, especially among young males (see Indicator 2.1 "Smoking and alcohol consumption at age 15").

Figure 2.7.3 shows the relationship between alcohol consumption in 2005 and deaths from liver cirrhosis in 2008. In general, countries with high levels of alcohol consumption tend to experience higher death rates from liver cirrhosis. In most EU countries, death rates from liver cirrhosis have fallen over the past two decades, following quite closely the overall reduction in alcohol consumption.

Definition and deviations

Alcohol consumption is defined as annual sales of pure alcohol in litres per person aged 15 years and over. The methodology to convert alcohol drinks to pure alcohol may differ across countries.

Italy reports consumption for the population 14 years and over, and Sweden for 16 years and over. In some countries (*e.g.* Luxembourg), national sales do not accurately reflect actual consumption by residents, since purchases by non-residents may create a significant gap between national sales and consumption.

2.7.1. Alcohol consumption among population aged 15 years and over

2008 (or nearest year available)   **Change per capita, 1980-2008**

	2008 (litres per capita)	Change per capita 1980-2008 (% change over period)
Turkey	1.4	-22
Malta	5.3	n.a.
Norway	6.8	28
Sweden	6.9	3
Iceland	7.3	70
Italy	8.1	-50
Greece	9.0	-32
Cyprus	9.3	50
Netherlands	9.6	-17
Slovak Republic	9.6	-34
Romania	9.7	-11
Germany	9.9	-30
Latvia	10.2	-22
Switzerland	10.2	-24
Finland	10.3	30
Belgium	10.7	-21
EU	**10.8**	**-13**
Poland	10.8	24
United Kingdom	10.8	15
Bulgaria	10.9	-2
Denmark	10.9	-7
Slovenia	10.9	n.a.
Portugal	11.4	-23
Spain	11.7	-36
Czech Republic	12.1	3
Ireland	12.4	29
Austria	12.5	-14
Lithuania	12.5	n.a.
France	12.6	-35
Hungary	12.6	-15
Estonia	14.0	n.a.
Luxembourg	15.5	16

Litres per capita

Source: OECD Health Data 2010; Eurostat Statistics Database; WHO (2010).

StatLink ⌨ http://dx.doi.org/10.1787/888932336559

2.7.2. Trends in alcohol consumption, selected EU countries, 1980-2008

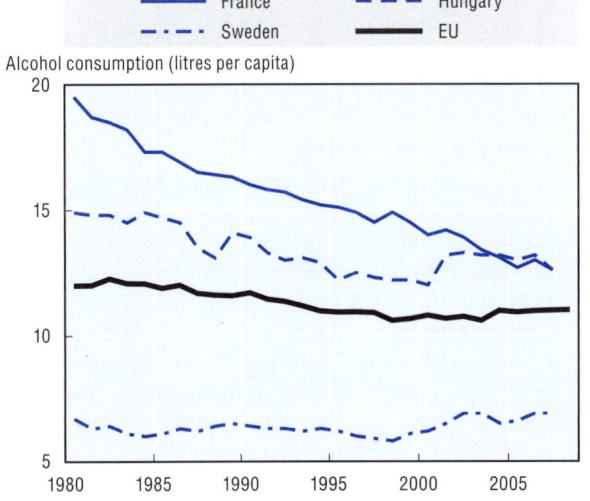

Source: OECD Health Data 2010; Eurostat Statistics Database; WHO (2010).

StatLink ⌨ http://dx.doi.org/10.1787/888932336578

2.7.3. Alcohol consumption, 2005 and chronic liver disease deaths, 2008 (or nearest year available)

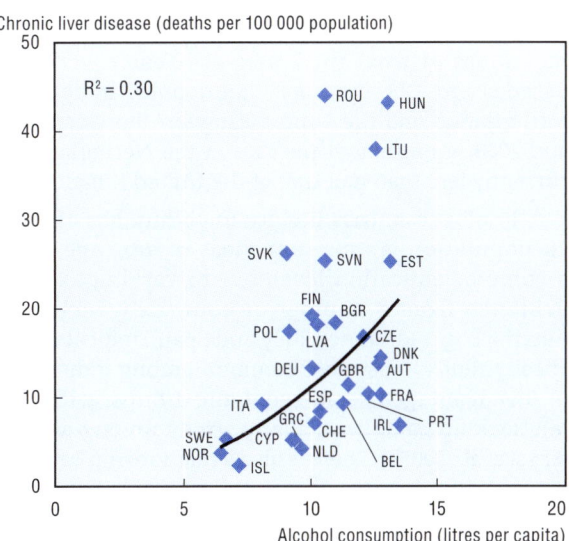

Source: OECD Health Data 2010; Eurostat Statistics Database; WHO (2010).

StatLink ⌨ http://dx.doi.org/10.1787/888932336597

The growth in overweight and obesity rates among adults is a major public health concern. Obesity is a known risk factor for numerous health problems, including hypertension, high cholesterol, diabetes, cardiovascular diseases, respiratory problems (asthma), musculoskeletal diseases (arthritis) and some forms of cancer. Mortality also increases sharply once the overweight threshold is crossed (OECD, 2010c).

More than half (50.1%) of the adult population in the European Union are overweight or obese. The prevalence of overweight and obesity among adults exceeds 50% in no less than 15 of 27 EU countries. In contrast, overweight and obesity rates are much lower in France, Italy and Switzerland, although rates are also increasing in these countries. The prevalence of obesity – which presents greater health risks than overweight – varies threefold among countries, from a low of less than 10% in Romania, Switzerland and Italy to over 20% in the United Kingdom, Ireland, Malta and Iceland (Figure 2.8.1). Across the European Union, 15.5% of the adult population is obese.

There is little difference in the average obesity rate of men and women in the European Union, with both at around 15% (Figure 2.8.1). However, there is some variation among individual countries, with men generally being more obese than women in Norway, Malta and Italy, whereas women are more obese in Latvia, Turkey and the Netherlands. The largest disparities in obesity between men and women were in Latvia, whereas there was little, if any difference in male and female obesity rates in the Czech Republic, Poland and Sweden.

The rate of obesity has more than doubled over the past 20 years in most EU countries for which data are available (Figure 2.8.2). The rapid increase occurred regardless of what the levels of obesity were two decades ago. Obesity more than doubled in both the Netherlands and the United Kingdom between 1988 and 2008, even though the rate in the Netherlands is currently less than half that of the United Kingdom.

In most countries the rise in obesity has affected all population groups regardless of sex, age, race, income or education level, but to varying extents. Evidence from a number of countries, including Austria, England, France, Italy and Spain, indicates that obesity tends to be more common among individuals in disadvantaged socio-economic groups, with this relationship being particularly strong among women (Sassi *et al.*, 2009b). There is also a relationship between the number of years spent in full-time education and obesity, with the most educated individuals displaying lower rates. Again, the gradient in obesity is stronger in women than in men (OECD, 2010c).

A number of behavioural and environmental factors have contributed to the rise in overweight and obesity rates in industrialised countries, including falling real prices of food and more time spent being physically inactive. Overweight and obesity has risen rapidly in children in recent decades, reaching double-figure rates in most EU countries (see Indicator 2.4).

Because obesity is associated with higher risks of chronic illnesses, it is linked to significant additional health care costs. There is a time lag between the onset of obesity and related health problems, suggesting that the rise in obesity over the past two decades will mean higher health care costs in the future. A recent study estimated that total costs linked to overweight and obesity in England in 2015 could increase by as much as 70% relative to 2007 and could be 2.4 times higher in 2025 (Foresight, 2007).

Definition and deviations

Overweight and obesity are defined as excessive weight presenting health risks because of the high proportion of body fat. The most frequently used measure is based on the body mass index (BMI), which is a single number that evaluates an individual's weight in relation to height (weight/height^2, with weight in kilograms and height in metres). Based on the WHO classification (WHO, 2000), adults with a BMI between 25 and 30 are defined as overweight, and those with a BMI over 30 as obese. This classification may not be suitable for all ethnic groups, who may have equivalent levels of risk at lower or higher BMI. The thresholds for adults are not suitable to measure overweight and obesity among children.

For most countries, overweight and obesity rates are self-reported through estimates of height and weight from population-based health interview surveys. The exceptions are Ireland, Luxembourg, the Slovak Republic (2008) and the United Kingdom, where estimates are derived from health examinations. These differences limit data comparability. Estimates from health examinations are generally higher and more reliable than from health interviews.

2.8.1. Obesity rates among adults, 2008 (or nearest year available)

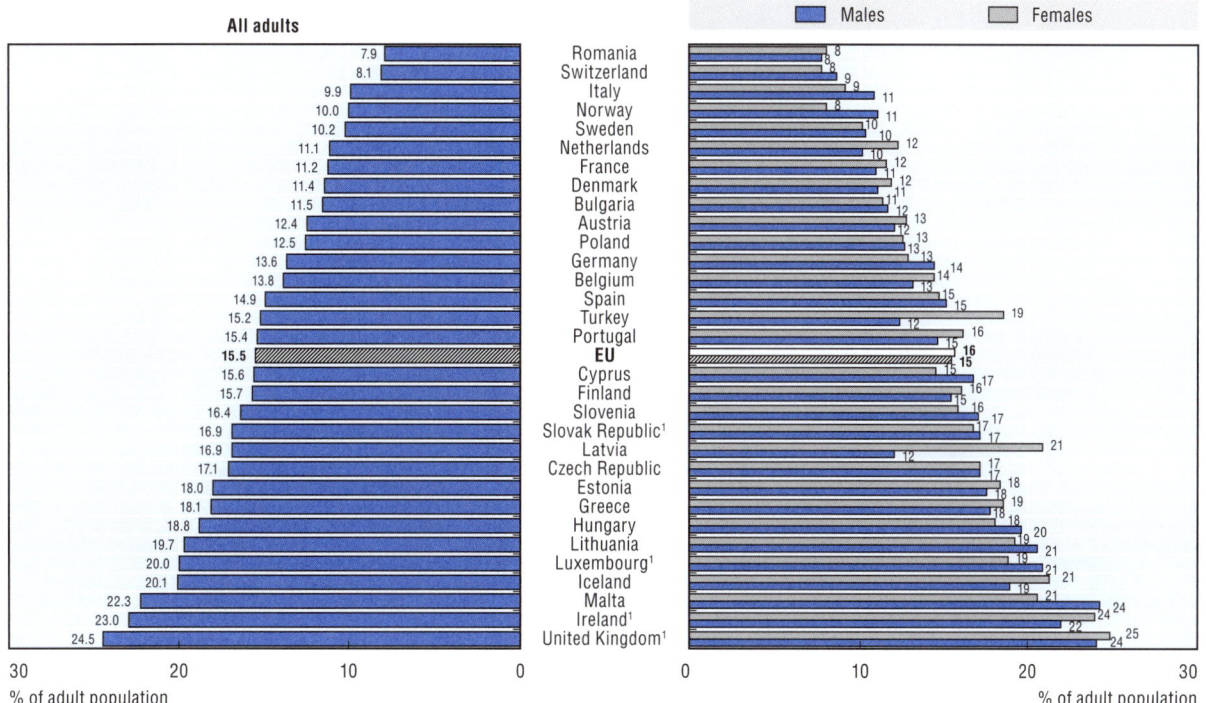

All adults

Males	Females

1. Ireland, Luxembourg, Slovak Republic and United Kingdom figures are based on health examination surveys, rather than health interview surveys.

Source: OECD Health Data 2010; Eurostat Statistics Database; WHO Global Infobase.

StatLink http://dx.doi.org/10.1787/888932336616

2.8.2. Increasing obesity rates among adults in EU countries

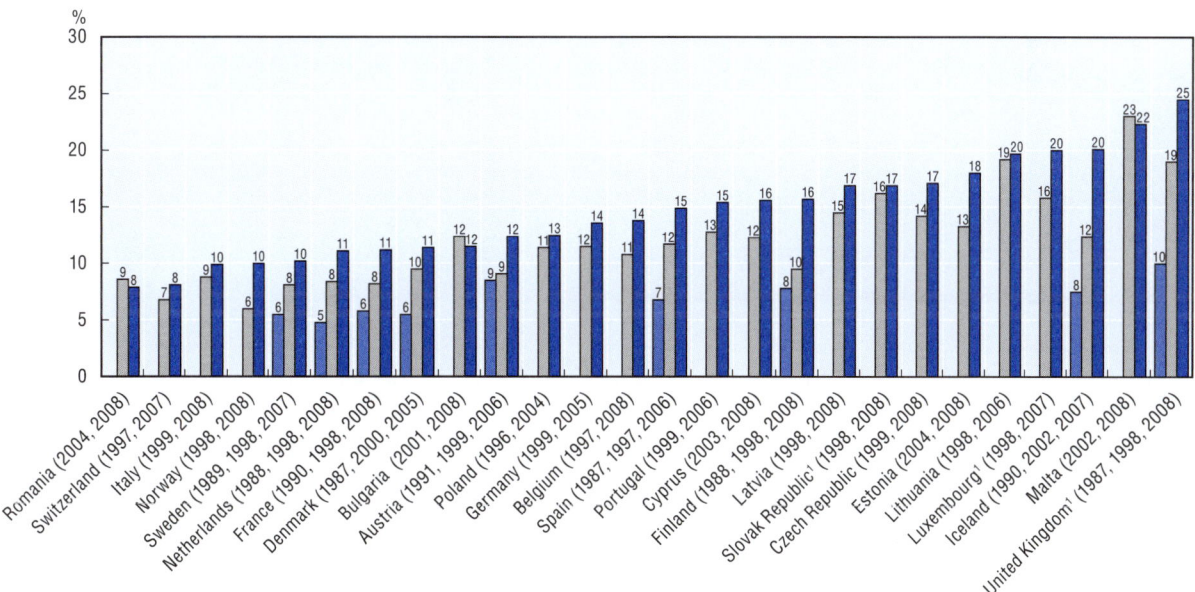

1. Luxembourg, Slovak Republic (2008) and United Kingdom figures are based on health examination surveys, rather than health interview surveys.

Source: OECD Health Data 2010; Eurostat Statistics Database; WHO Global Infobase.

StatLink http://dx.doi.org/10.1787/888932336635

Chapter 3

Health Care Resources, Services and Outcomes

Access to high-quality services depends crucially on the size, skill mix, geographic distribution and productivity of the health workforce. Health workers, and in particular doctors and nurses, are the cornerstone of health systems.

In 2008, Greece had, by far, the highest number of doctors per capita, with six doctors per 1 000 population, nearly twice the EU average. Following Greece were Austria, Italy and Norway, with four doctors or more per 1 000 population. The number of doctors per capita was the lowest in Turkey, followed by Poland and Romania. Doctor numbers are also relatively low in the United Kingdom and Finland (Figure 3.1.1).

Since 2000, the number of physicians per capita has increased in all European countries, except the Slovak Republic. On average across EU countries, physician density grew at a rate of 1.5% per year, rising from 3.0 doctors per 1 000 population to 3.3. The growth rate was particularly rapid in Turkey, which started from the lowest level in 2000, thereby narrowing the gap with other countries.

The number of doctors also increased rapidly in Ireland, rising by nearly 50% (from 2.2 per 1 000 population in 2000 to 3.2 in 2008). A large part of this increase is due to the recruitment of foreign-trained physicians. The share of foreign-trained physicians in Ireland more than tripled during this period, rising from 11% of all physicians in 2000 to 35% in 2008 (OECD and WHO, 2010). There has also been a substantial rise in the number of students graduating from medical schools in Ireland (OECD, 2010a).

A similar pattern has been observed in the United Kingdom, where the number of doctors went up from 2.0 per 1 000 population in 2000 to 2.6 in 2008, an increase of 30%. The number of new registrations of foreign-trained doctors in the United Kingdom increased to 2003 when it peaked at about 14 000, but has declined since then to just over 5 000 in 2008 (OECD and WHO, 2010). At the same time, the number of new graduates from medical schools in the United Kingdom increased, from about 4 600 in 2003 to 5 600 in 2008, gradually exceeding the number of new registrations of foreign-trained physicians.

In contrast, in France and Italy there was virtually no growth. Following the reduction in the number of new entrants in medical schools during the 1980s and 1990s, the number of doctors per capita in Italy peaked in 2002, and has declined since then. In France, the number peaked in 2005, and the decline is expected to continue to 2020 (DREES, 2009).

In nearly all countries, the balance between general practitioners and specialists has changed over past decades, with the number of specialists increasing much more rapidly than generalists. As a result, there are more specialists than generalists in all countries, except Romania and Portugal (Figure 3.1.2). A number of reasons explain this trend. There may be less interest in the traditional mode of practice of general/family practitioner and the workload and constraints attached to it. In addition, in many countries, there is a growing remuneration gap between generalists and specialists (Fujisawa and Lafortune, 2008). The slow or negative growth in the number of generalists per capita raises concerns about access to primary care for certain population groups. In response to this shortage, many countries are considering ways to improve the attractiveness of general practice as well as the development of new roles for other health care providers, such as nurses (Delamaire and Lafortune, 2010).

Definition and deviations

Practising physicians are defined as doctors who are providing care directly to patients. In some countries, the numbers also include doctors working in administration, management, academic and research positions ("professionally active" physicians), adding another 5-10% of doctors. Ireland, the Netherlands and Portugal report all physicians entitled to practice, resulting in an over-estimation.

Not all countries are able to report all physicians as generalists or specialists, and in some countries (e.g. the Netherlands), most physicians are not reported in either of these two broad categories. In some countries, data on medical specialty may not be available for interns/residents (physicians in training) or for those working in private practice.

3.1.1. Practising physicians per 1 000 population

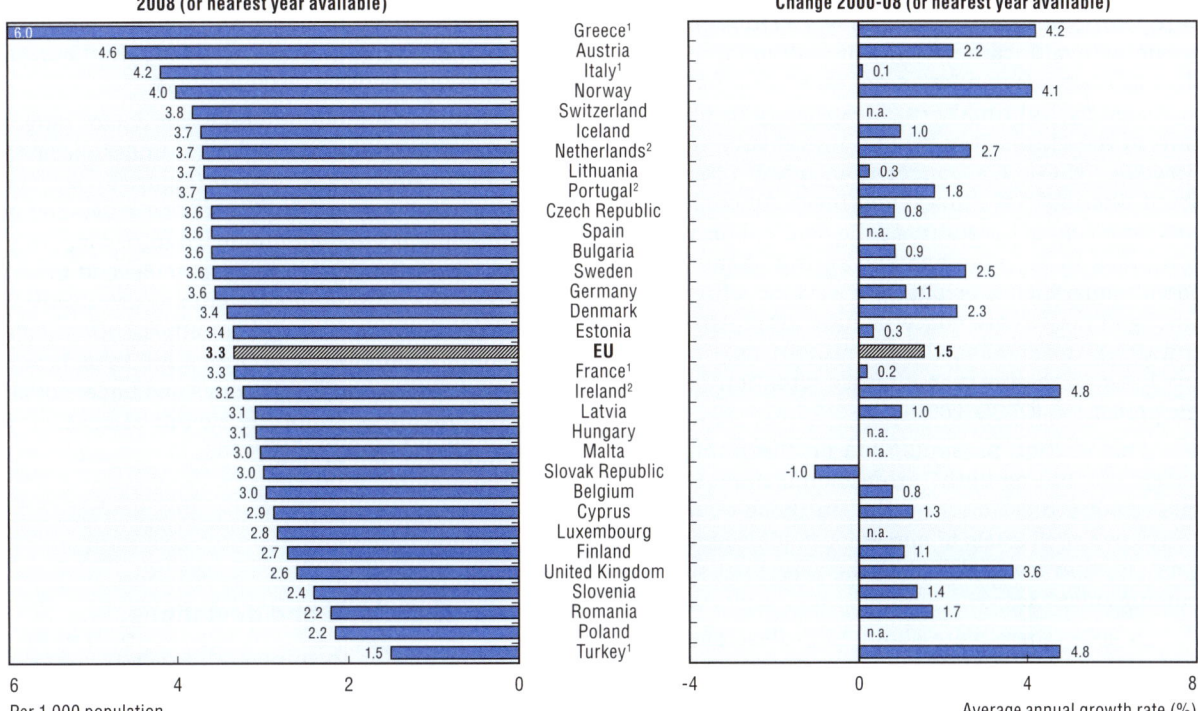

2008 (or nearest year available)   **Change 2000-08 (or nearest year available)**

	2008 value	Change %
Greece[1]	6.0	4.2
Austria	4.6	2.2
Italy[1]	4.2	0.1
Norway	4.0	4.1
Switzerland	3.8	n.a.
Iceland	3.7	1.0
Netherlands[2]	3.7	2.7
Lithuania	3.7	0.3
Portugal[2]	3.7	1.8
Czech Republic	3.6	0.8
Spain	3.6	n.a.
Bulgaria	3.6	0.9
Sweden	3.6	2.5
Germany	3.6	1.1
Denmark	3.4	2.3
Estonia	3.4	0.3
EU	**3.3**	**1.5**
France[1]	3.3	0.2
Ireland[2]	3.2	4.8
Latvia	3.1	1.0
Hungary	3.1	n.a.
Malta	3.0	n.a.
Slovak Republic	3.0	-1.0
Belgium	3.0	0.8
Cyprus	2.9	1.3
Luxembourg	2.8	n.a.
Finland	2.7	1.1
United Kingdom	2.6	3.6
Slovenia	2.4	1.4
Romania	2.2	1.7
Poland	2.2	n.a.
Turkey[1]	1.5	4.8

Per 1 000 population   Average annual growth rate (%)

1. Data include not only physicians providing direct care to patients, but also those working in the health sector as managers, educators, researchers, etc. (adding another 5-10% of doctors).
2. Data refer to all physicians who are licensed to practice.

Source: OECD Health Data 2010; Eurostat Statistics Database.

StatLink http://dx.doi.org/10.1787/888932336654

3.1.2. General practitioners, specialists and other physicians as a share of total physicians, 2008 (or nearest year available)

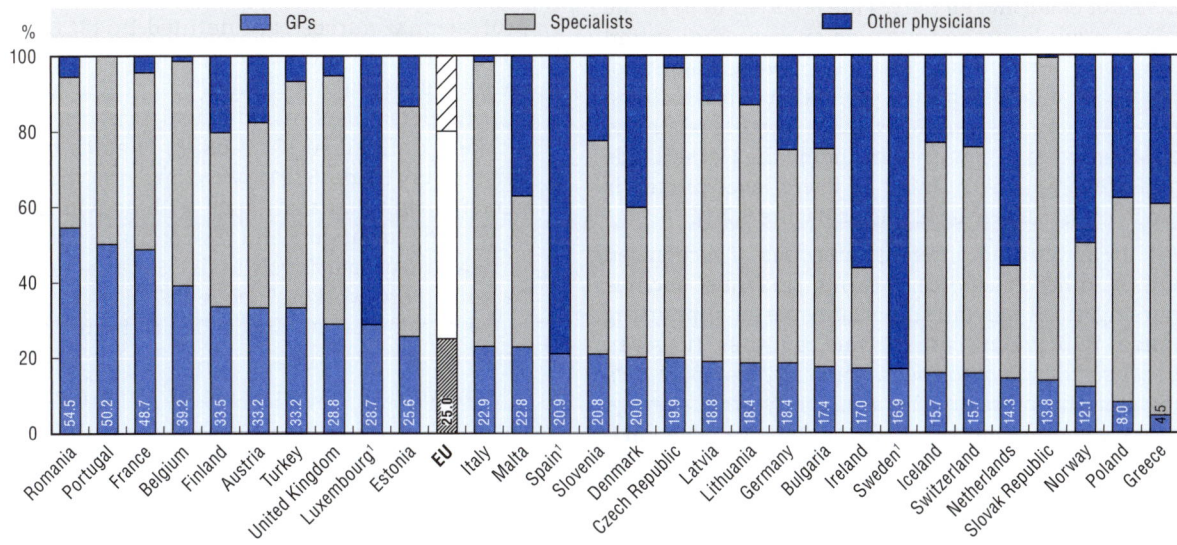

GPs   Specialists   Other physicians

Country	GPs %
Romania	54.5
Portugal	50.2
France	48.7
Belgium	39.2
Finland	33.5
Austria	33.2
Turkey	33.2
United Kingdom	28.8
Luxembourg[1]	28.7
Estonia	25.6
EU	25.0
Italy	22.9
Malta	22.8
Spain[1]	20.9
Slovenia	20.8
Denmark	20.0
Czech Republic	19.9
Latvia	18.8
Lithuania	18.4
Germany	18.4
Bulgaria	17.4
Ireland	17.0
Sweden[1]	16.9
Iceland	15.7
Switzerland	15.7
Netherlands	14.3
Slovak Republic	13.8
Norway	12.1
Poland	8.0
Greece	4.5

Note: Specialists include paediatricians, obstetricians/gynaecologists, psychiatrists, medical specialists and surgical specialists. Other physicians include interns/residents if not reported in the field in which they are training, and doctors not elsewhere classified.
1. Data are not available for specialists.

Source: OECD Health Data 2010; Eurostat Statistics Database.

StatLink http://dx.doi.org/10.1787/888932336673

Nurses are usually the most numerous health profession, outnumbering physicians in most European countries. Nurses play a critical role in providing health care not only in traditional settings such as hospitals and long-term care institutions but increasingly in primary care (especially in offering care to the chronically ill) and in patients' homes. However, there are concerns in many countries about shortages of nurses, and these concerns may well intensify in the future as the demand for nurses continues to increase and the ageing of the "baby boom" generation precipitates a wave of retirements among nurses. These concerns have prompted many countries to increase the training of new nurses combined with efforts to increase retention rates in the profession (OECD, 2008b).

This section presents data on the number of nurses, including both "professional nurses" and "associate professional nurses" in those countries where two such levels of nurses exist. It also provides data on other lower-skilled caring personnel such as nursing aides.

In 2008, there were about 15 professional and associate professional nurses per 1 000 population in Finland, Iceland, Ireland and Switzerland, and slightly fewer in Denmark and Norway. Turkey had the fewest nurses, followed by Greece, Bulgaria and Cyprus, with all these countries having fewer than five nurses per 1 000 population.

The mix between different categories of nurses varies widely across European countries. In some countries such as France, Portugal and Poland, a lower-level category of "associate professional nurses" does not exist, and all nurses are reported to be at the same level. In other countries such as the United Kingdom, Germany and Austria, the vast majority of nurses are considered to be professional nurses, but a minority are considered to be at a lower-level. In yet another group of countries including the Netherlands and Slovenia, the number of lower-level nurses is greater than higher-level nurses (Figure 3.2.1).

In addition to different categories of recognised nurses, other categories of caring personnel such as nursing aides play an important role in supporting nurses in providing care in some countries. However, because these personnel are usually not part of a registered profession, the availability and coverage of data is more limited. Based on the available data, the number of such additional caring personnel is the highest in the Netherlands, Norway and Denmark. In the Netherlands and France, there are in fact more caring personnel than nurses.

Since 2000, the number of nurses per capita has increased in all European countries, except in Lithuania and the Slovak Republic. The increase was particularly large in Portugal and Spain, where the number of nurses per population increased by 45% and 33% respectively. In France and Switzerland, there was also a fairly large increase in the supply of nurses, rising by 15-20% between 2000 and 2008.

In 2008, the number of nurses per doctor ranged from about six in Ireland and Finland to under one nurse per doctor in Greece and Turkey (Figure 3.2.2). The average across European countries is over two-and-a-half nurses per doctor, with many countries reporting between two to four nurses per doctor. Beyond Greece and Turkey, the nurse-to-doctor ratio is also relatively low in other southern European countries, such as Italy, Spain, Portugal and Cyprus. In Greece and Italy, there is evidence of an over-supply of doctors and under-supply of nurses, resulting in an inefficient allocation of resources (OECD, 2009; Chaloff, 2008).

Definition and deviations

The data refer to nurses and other caring personnel providing direct care to patients, although in some countries they also include nurses working in management, research and other roles. This adds another 5-10% to nursing numbers.

"Professional nurses" are defined by ISCO-08 code 2221, and include categories of nurses such as registered nurses, clinical nurses, nurse anaesthetists, nurse practitioners, public health nurses, and specialist nurses. "Associate professional nurses" are defined by ISCO-08 code 3221, and include categories of nurses such as "enrolled nurses" and "practical nurses". "Caring personnel" includes two categories of workers defined in ISCO-08: 1) "health care assistants" (code 5321) who "provide direct personal care and assistance with activities of daily living to patients and residents in a variety of health care settings"; and 2) "home-based personal care workers" (code 5322), including home care aides, nursing aides at home, and personal care providers.

Midwives are usually excluded from nurses. However, about half of European countries report midwives together with nurses, as they are considered specialist nurses.

Austria reports only nurses working in hospitals. The data for Germany does not include nurses who have three years of education and are providing services for the elderly.

3.2.1. Professional nurses, associate professional nurses and caring personnel per 1 000 population, 2008 (or nearest year available)

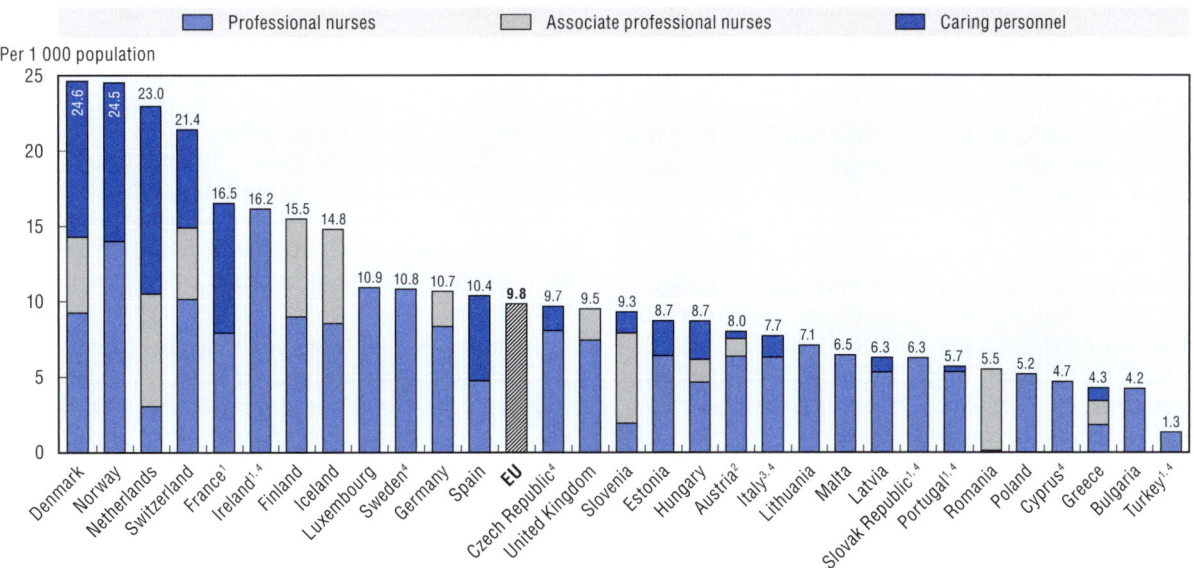

1. Data include not only nurses providing direct care to patients, but also those working in the health sector as managers, educators, researchers, etc. (adding another 5-10% of nurses).
2. Austria reports only nurses employed in hospitals.
3. In Italy, data refer to all nurses who are licensed to practice.
4. The breakdown between professional and associate professional nurses is not available.

Source: OECD Health Data 2010; Eurostat Statistics Database.

StatLink http://dx.doi.org/10.1787/888932336692

3.2.2. Ratio of nurses to physicians, 2008 (or nearest year available)

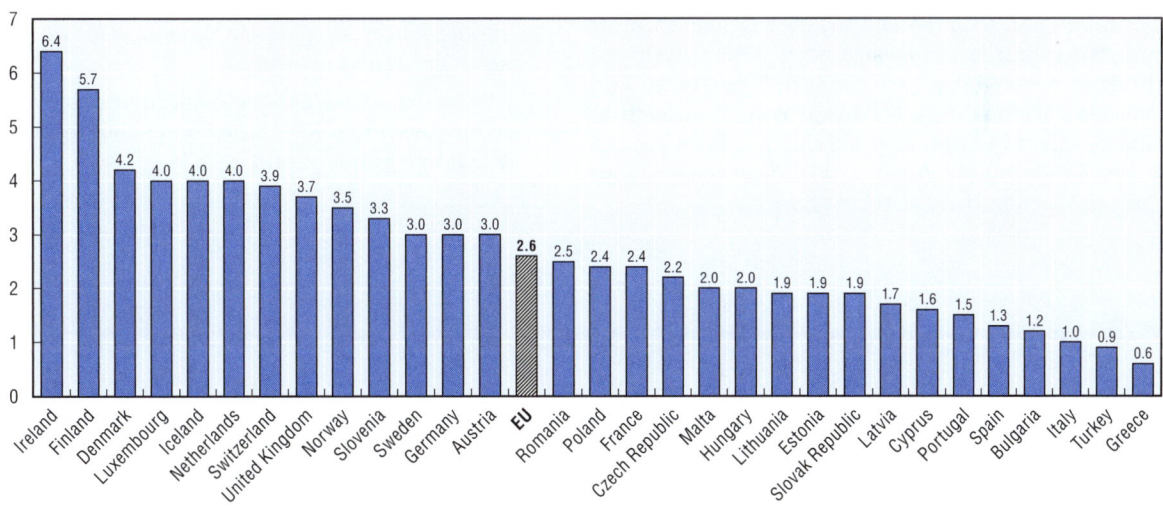

Note: Nurses only include professional and associate professional nurses and exclude other caring personnel.

Source: OECD Health Data 2010; Eurostat Statistics Database.

StatLink http://dx.doi.org/10.1787/888932336711

Childhood vaccination continues to be one of the most cost-effective public health interventions. All European countries, or in some cases sub-national jurisdictions, have established vaccination programmes based on their interpretation of the risks and benefits of each vaccine.

Vaccination against pertussis (often administered in connection with vaccination against diphtheria and tetanus) and measles is part of almost all programmes. Reviews of the evidence supporting the efficacy of vaccines against these diseases have concluded that the respective vaccines are safe and highly effective. In the European Union, the gradual take-up of the measles vaccine has meant that measles incidence is around twenty times lower than the rate of the early 1990s (see Indicator 1.11), although outbreak can still occur.

A vaccination for hepatitis B has been available since 1982 and is considered to be 95% effective in preventing infection and its chronic consequences, such as cirrhosis and liver cancer. In 2004, it was estimated that over 350 million people were chronically infected with the hepatitis B virus worldwide and at risk of serious illness and death (WHO, 2009a). In 2007, more than 170 countries had already begun to follow the WHO recommendation to incorporate hepatitis B vaccine as an integral part of their national infant immunisation programme.

Figures 3.3.1 and 3.3.2 demonstrate that the overall vaccination of children against pertussis (including diphtheria and tetanus) and measles is high in most European countries. On average, about 95% of 2-year-old children receive the recommended pertussis and measles vaccination, a level that is high enough to provide effective immunity. Vaccination rates are the lowest in Malta and Austria, with less than 85% of children vaccinated against these diseases.

Figure 3.3.3 shows that the average percentage of children aged 2 years vaccinated for hepatitis B across countries with national programmes is also over 95%. However, some European countries do not currently require children to be vaccinated by age 2, or do not have routine programmes, and consequently the rates for these countries are significantly lower. For example, in Denmark and Sweden, vaccination against hepatitis B is not an obligatory part of vaccination programmes, and is only recommended to specific risk groups. In France, hepatitis B vaccination remains controversial, given ongoing speculation over possible side effects.

Figure 1.11.3 in Chapter 1 indicates that the incidence of hepatitis B is low in the majority of European countries, at less than 2 per 100 000 population. However, in Iceland, Bulgaria, Turkey, Austria, Latvia and Romania, the rates are more than two times the EU average.

Definition and deviation

Vaccination rates reflect the percentage of children at age 1 or 2 receiving the respective vaccination. Childhood vaccination policies differ across countries. Some countries administer combination vaccines (*e.g.* DTP for diphtheria, tetanus and pertussis) while others administer the vaccinations separately. Schedules for administering vaccines also differ.

Some countries ascertain vaccinations based on surveys and others based on encounter data, which may influence the results.

3.3.1. Vaccination rates for pertussis, children aged 2, 2008 (or nearest year available)

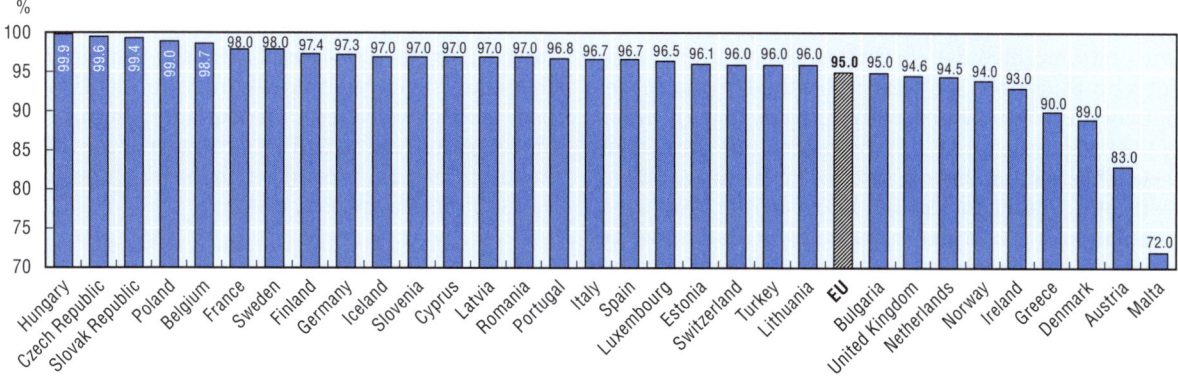

Source: OECD Health Data 2010; WHO vaccine-preventable diseases: monitoring system 2010 global summary.

StatLink ⟐⟐⟐ http://dx.doi.org/10.1787/888932336730

3.3.2. Vaccination rates for measles, children aged 2, 2008 (or nearest year available)

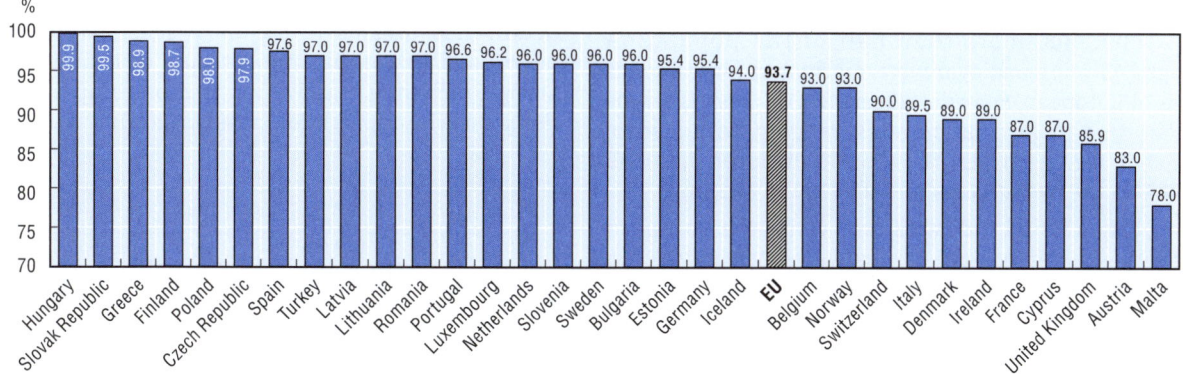

Source: OECD Health Data 2010; WHO vaccine-preventable diseases: monitoring system 2010 global summary.

StatLink ⟐⟐⟐ http://dx.doi.org/10.1787/888932336749

3.3.3. Vaccination rates for hepatitis B, children aged 2, 2008 (or nearest year available)

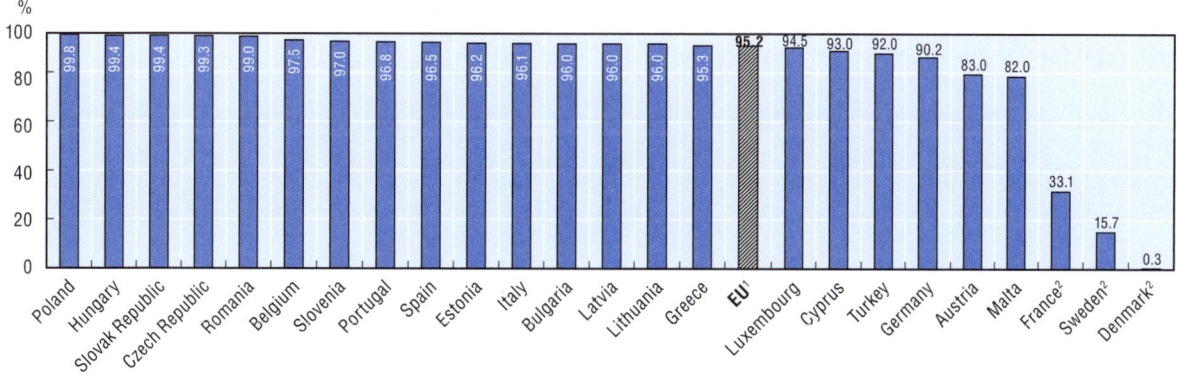

1. EU average only includes countries with required or routine immunisation.
2. In France, Sweden and Denmark, vaccination for hepatitis B is not required or routinely provided.

Source: OECD Health Data 2010; WHO vaccine-preventable diseases: monitoring system 2010 global summary.

StatLink ⟐⟐⟐ http://dx.doi.org/10.1787/888932336768

Influenza is a common infectious disease worldwide and affects persons of all ages. Most people with the illness recover quickly, but elderly people and those with chronic medical conditions are at higher risk for complications and even death. For example, between 2000 and 2008, influenza along with other acute upper respiratory infections accounted for about 44 000 hospitalisations per year in France and 77 000 in Germany. The impact of influenza on the employed population is substantial, even though most influenza morbidity and mortality occurs among the elderly and those with chronic conditions (*e.g.* 85-90% of people who die from influenza in France and Germany are over 65 years of age).

Immunisation against seasonal influenza (or flu) for older people has become increasingly widespread in many European countries over the past decade. Influenza vaccination for patients with chronic conditions and other at-risk groups is also strongly recommended in many countries.

In 2008, more than half of the population aged 65 years and over were vaccinated for influenza in 14 European countries (Figure 3.4.1). There is a wide variation in vaccination rates, ranging from lows of 21% in the Czech Republic and 26% in Slovenia, to over 75% in the Netherlands and the United Kingdom.

Figure 3.4.2 indicates that while the European average increased markedly between 1998 and 2003, it remained relatively stable between 2003 and 2008. From 2003, some countries marginally increased their coverage whereas others reduced it, most notably in countries which were already below the EU average, such as Slovenia, the Slovak Republic and Hungary.

A number of factors contributed to the rise in influenza immunisation rates in most European countries over the past decade, including greater acceptance of preventive health services by patients and practitioners, improved public health insurance coverage for vaccines, and wider delivery by health care providers other than physicians. However, a number of barriers need to be overcome in some countries if they wish to increase their coverage rates further. For example, possible reasons put forward for the relatively low vaccination rates in Austria include poor public awareness, inadequate insurance coverage of related costs, and lack of consensus within the Austrian medical profession about the importance of vaccination (Kunze *et al.*, 2007).

New types of influenza, such as the H1N1 "swine flu", have emerged in recent years and prompted rapid responses to contain the pandemic. While symptoms of the H1N1 influenza are mild in most people, a minority have suffered severe disease with some dying from it. The majority of those people who have suffered severely from the disease have other chronic medical conditions such as asthma or heart disease. But there have also been cases of people who became severely ill without any underlying condition (European Commission, 2010c). A series of public health measures used to combat seasonal flu have been used to combat new strains of influenza in Europe, including massive vaccination campaigns for risk groups (European Commission, 2010c).

Definitions and deviations

Influenza vaccination rate refers to the number of people aged 65 and older who have received an annual influenza vaccination, divided by the total number of people over 65 years of age. The main limitation in terms of data comparability arises from the use of different data sources, whether survey or programme, which are susceptible to different types of errors and biases.

3.4.1. Influenza vaccination coverage, population aged 65 and over, 2008 (or nearest year available)

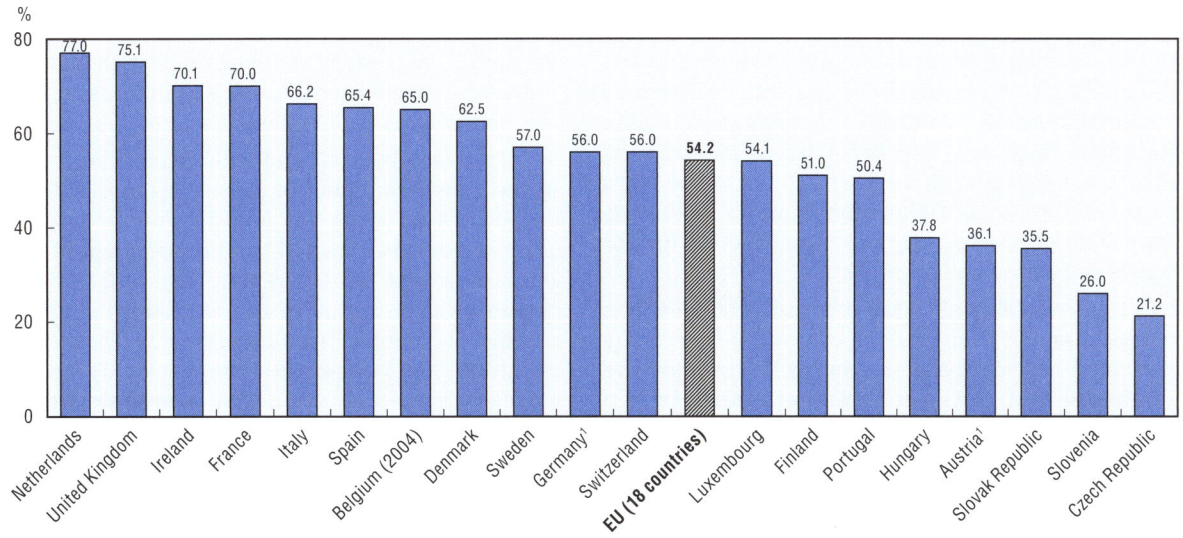

1. Population aged 60 and over.
Source: OECD Health Data 2010.

StatLink ⊕ http://dx.doi.org/10.1787/888932336787

3.4.2. Vaccination rates for influenza, population aged 65 and over, 1998-2008 (or nearest year available)

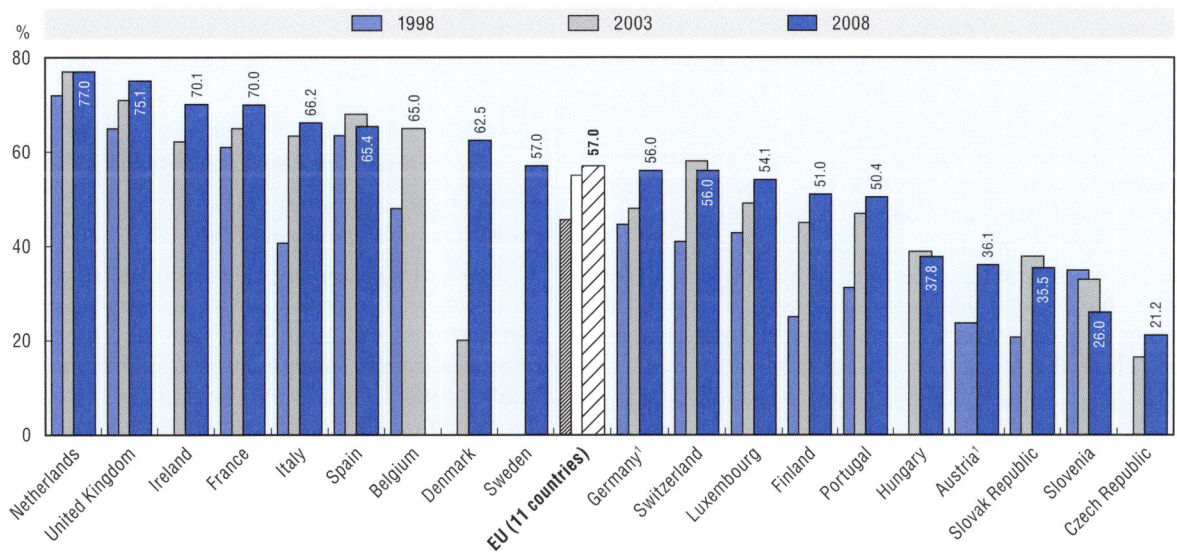

1. Population aged 60 and over.
Source: OECD Health Data 2010.

StatLink ⊕ http://dx.doi.org/10.1787/888932336806

New medical technologies are improving diagnosis and treatment, but they are also increasing health spending. This section presents data on the availability and use of two diagnostic technologies: computed tomography (CT) scanners and magnetic resonance imaging (MRI) units. CT scanners and MRI units help physicians diagnose a range of conditions by producing images of internal organs and structures of the body. Unlike conventional radiography and CT scanning, newer imaging technology used in MRI units do not expose patients to ionising radiation.

The availability of CT scanners and MRI units has increased rapidly in most European countries over the past two decades. For example, in the Netherlands, the number of MRI units per capita multiplied by ten between 1990 and 2008, while the number of CT scanners also increased. Similarly, in Italy, the number of MRI scanners per capita multiplied by five between 1997 and 2007, and the number of CT scanners doubled.

In 2008, Greece had the highest number of MRI and CT scanners per capita (together with Cyprus for CT scanners). Switzerland, Iceland, Italy and Austria also had significantly more MRI and CT scanners than the EU average (Figures 3.5.1 and 3.5.2). However, the number of MRI and CT scanners in all European countries remains much lower than in Japan and the United States (OECD, 2010a). The number of MRI units and CT scanners per population were the lowest in Romania and Hungary.

There is no general guideline regarding an ideal number of CT scanners or MRI units per population. However, if there are too few such items of equipment, this may lead to access problems, either in terms of geographic proximity or waiting times. On the other hand, if there are too many, this may result in an overuse of these costly diagnostic procedures, with little if any benefits to patients.

Data on the use of these diagnostic equipment are available only for a smaller group of countries. Based on this more limited country coverage, the number of CT and MRI exams per capita is the highest in Greece, consistent with the fact that Greece also has the highest number of these two types of scanners (Figures 3.5.3 and 3.5.4). The number of CT and MRI exams per capita is also above average in Belgium, Luxembourg and Iceland. It is the lowest in the Slovak Republic and Czech Republic, as well as in the Netherlands for CT exams.

In Greece, most CT and MRI scanners are installed in the growing number of private diagnostic centres, and only a minority are found in public hospitals. There is no regulation concerning the purchase of MRI units in Greece, while the purchase of CT scanners requires a licence that is granted following a review based on a criteria of population density. There are also no guidelines concerning the use of CT and MRI scanners (Paris et al., 2010). The current situation has led the Greek Ministry of Health and Social Solidarity to establish an expert's committee to review regulations and propose new criteria for the purchase of CT and MRI scanners.

Many other European countries are also examining ways to promote more rational purchase and use of such diagnostic technologies (OECD, 2010b). In the United Kingdom, the National Institute for Health and Clinical Excellence has recently set up a Diagnostics Advisory Committee to evaluate and make recommendations for the appropriate use of diagnostic technologies within the NHS in England (NICE, 2009).

Definition and deviations

The figures relate to the number of CT and MRI scanners per million population.

The data generally cover the equipment installed in hospitals and ambulatory settings, with the exception of Belgium, Germany and Spain where the equipment outside hospitals is not included, and France where only a small number of equipment in ambulatory settings is included. In the United Kingdom, the data refer only to scanners in the public sector.

3.5.1. Number of MRI units, 2008 (or nearest year available)

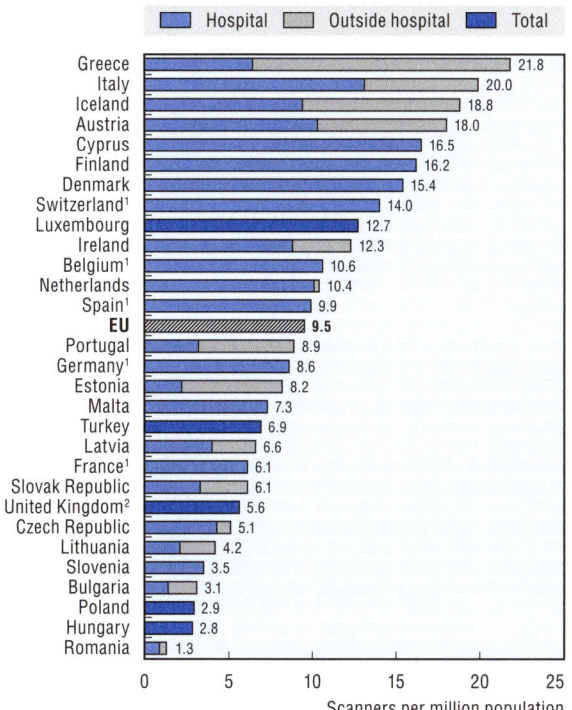

Note: The EU average does not include countries which only report equipment in hospital.
1. Data for equipment outside hospital are not available.
2. In the United Kingdom, any equipment in the private sector is not included in the data.

Source: OECD Health Data 2010; Eurostat Statistics Database.

StatLink http://dx.doi.org/10.1787/888932336825

3.5.2. Number of CT scanners, 2008 (or nearest year available)

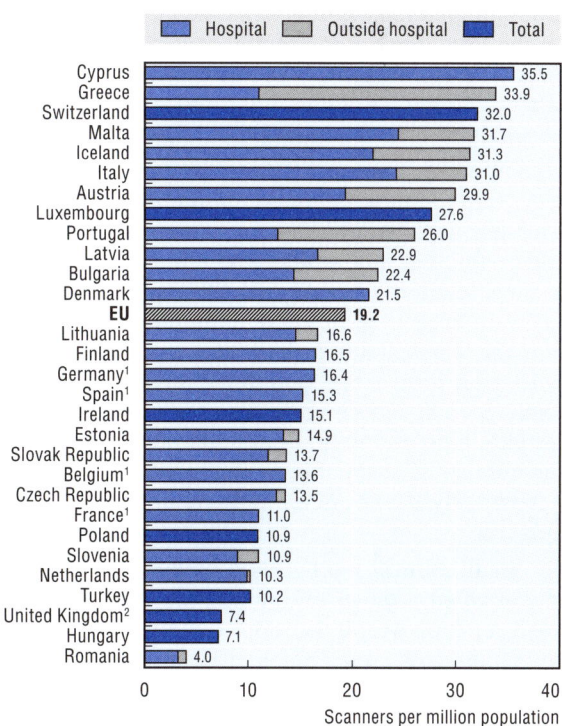

Note: The EU average does not include countries which only report equipment in hospital.
1. Data for equipment outside hospital are not available.
2. In the United Kingdom, any equipment in the private sector is not included in the data.

Source: OECD Health Data 2010; Eurostat Statistics Database.

StatLink http://dx.doi.org/10.1787/888932336844

3.5.3. Number of MRI exams, 2008 (or nearest year available)

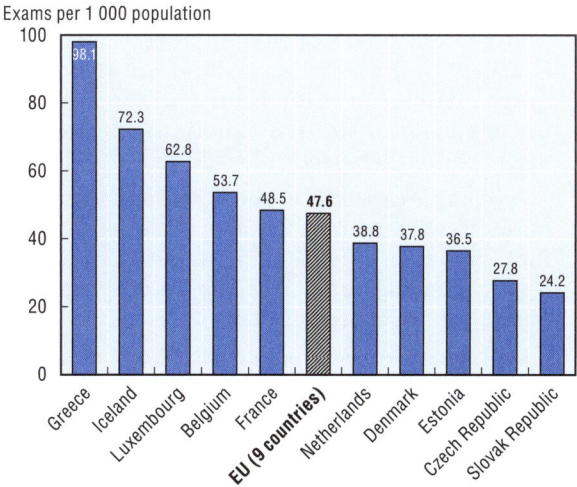

Source: OECD Health Data 2010.

StatLink http://dx.doi.org/10.1787/888932336863

3.5.4. Number of CT exams, 2008 (or nearest year available)

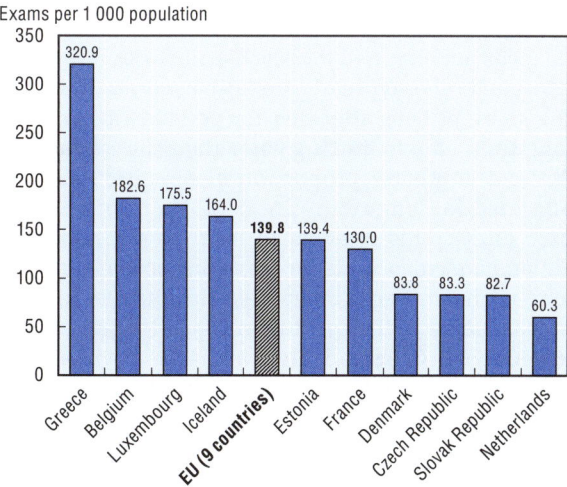

Source: OECD Health Data 2010.

StatLink http://dx.doi.org/10.1787/888932336882

The number of hospital beds provides an indication of the resources available for delivering services to in-patients in hospitals. This section presents data on the total number of hospital beds, including those allocated for curative, psychiatric, long-term and other types of care. It does not capture the capacity of hospitals to furnish same-day emergency or elective interventions.

Over the past 15 years, the number of hospital beds per population has decreased in all European countries. On average across EU countries, the number fell from 7.3 beds per 1 000 population in 1995 to 5.7 in 2008 (Figure 3.6.1). This reduction in the number of hospital beds has been accompanied by a reduction in average length of stays in hospitals (Indicator 3.8) and, in some countries, a reduction in hospital admissions (Indicator 3.7). The reduction in the number of hospital beds per population has been particularly pronounced in Latvia, Lithuania and Bulgaria.

In all countries, progress in medical technologies has enabled a move to day-surgery and a reduced need for long hospitalisation. In addition, in many countries, cost-containment policies over the past decade or so have targeted the hospital sector, as it remains the largest health spending category in most European countries.

In 2008, Germany and Austria had the highest number of hospital beds per capita, with about 8 beds per 1 000 population (Figure 3.6.1). The high supply of hospital beds in these two countries is associated with a large number of hospital admissions/discharges, as well as long average length of stays in Germany. Turkey had the lowest number of beds per capita, followed by Spain, the United Kingdom and Portugal.

Two-thirds of hospital beds are allocated for curative care on average across EU countries. The rest of the beds are allocated for psychiatric (14%), long-term (10%) and other types of care (8%). In some countries, the share of beds allocated for psychiatric care and long-term care is much greater than the average. In Finland, a greater proportion of hospital beds are allocated for long-term care (35%) than for curative care (30%). This is because local governments in Finland are responsible for managing both health and long-term care services, and use hospitals to provide at least some of the institution-based long-term care (OECD, 2005). In Ireland, just over half of hospital beds are allocated for acute care, with 30% devoted to long-term care (Figure 3.6.2).

The share of beds in private for-profit hospitals has increased in some countries over the past few years, while it has remained stable in others. In Germany, the share increased from 23% of all beds in 2002 to 29% in 2008, accompanied by a decline in the share of beds in public hospitals from 44% to 41%. The remaining 30% were beds in private not-for-profit hospitals, whose share also declined slightly. In Austria also, the share of beds in private for-profit hospitals has increased over the past decade, from 7% in 1995 to just over 10% in 2008, although the vast majority of beds continue to be in publically-owned hospitals. In France, the allocation of beds in public and private hospitals has remained fairly stable since 1997, with about 65% of beds located in public hospitals, 15% in private not-for-profit hospitals, and the remaining 20% in private for-profit hospitals (OECD, 2010a).

In several countries, the reduction in the overall number of hospital beds has been accompanied by an increase in their occupancy rates. Since 1995, the occupancy rate of curative care beds increased significantly in Ireland, Italy, Norway and Switzerland (OECD, 2010a).

Definition and deviations

Hospital beds are defined as all beds that are regularly maintained and staffed and are immediately available for use. They include beds in general hospitals, mental health and substance abuse hospitals, and other specialty hospitals. Beds in nursing and residential care facilities are excluded.

Curative care beds are beds accommodating patients where the principal intent is to do one or more of the following: manage labour (obstetric), cure non-mental illness or provide definitive treatment of injury, perform surgery, relieve symptoms of non-mental illness or injury (excluding palliative care), reduce severity of non-mental illness or injury, protect against exacerbation and/or complication of non-mental illness and/or injury which could threaten life or normal functions, perform diagnostic or therapeutic procedures.

Psychiatric care beds are beds accommodating patients with mental health problems. They include beds in psychiatric departments of general hospitals, and all beds in mental health and substance abuse hospitals.

Long-term care beds are hospital beds accommodating patients requiring long-term care due to chronic impairments and a reduced degree of independence in activities of daily living. They include beds in long-term care departments of general hospitals, beds for long-term care in specialty hospitals, and beds for palliative care.

3.6.1. Hospital beds per 1 000 population, 1995 and 2008 (or nearest year available)

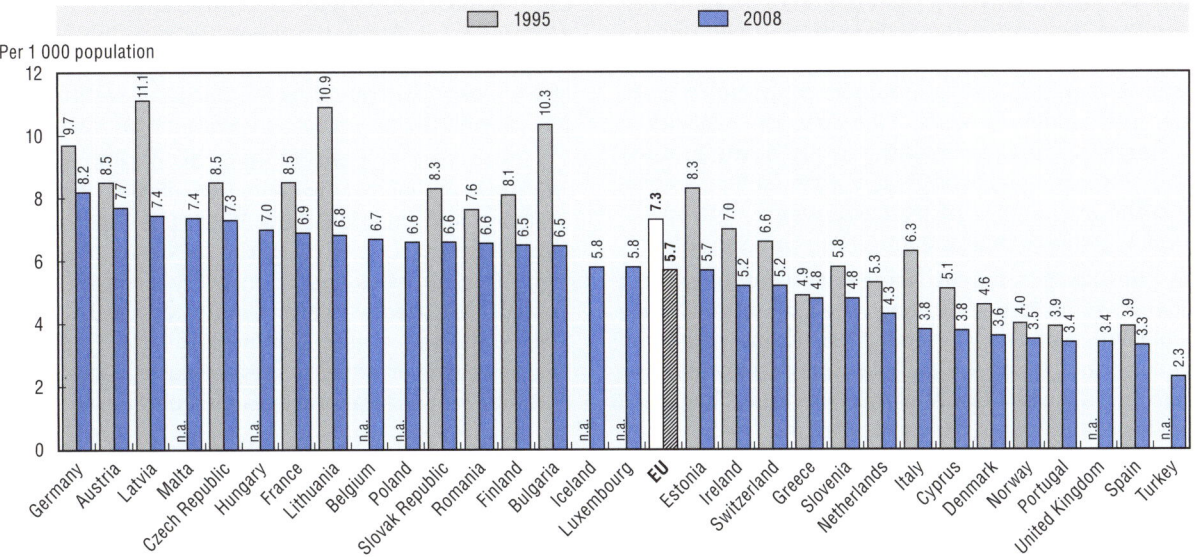

Source: OECD Health Data 2010; Eurostat Statistics Database.

StatLink http://dx.doi.org/10.1787/888932336901

3.6.2. Hospital beds by function of health care, 2008 (or nearest year available)

Countries ranked by declining order of hospital beds per 1 000 population

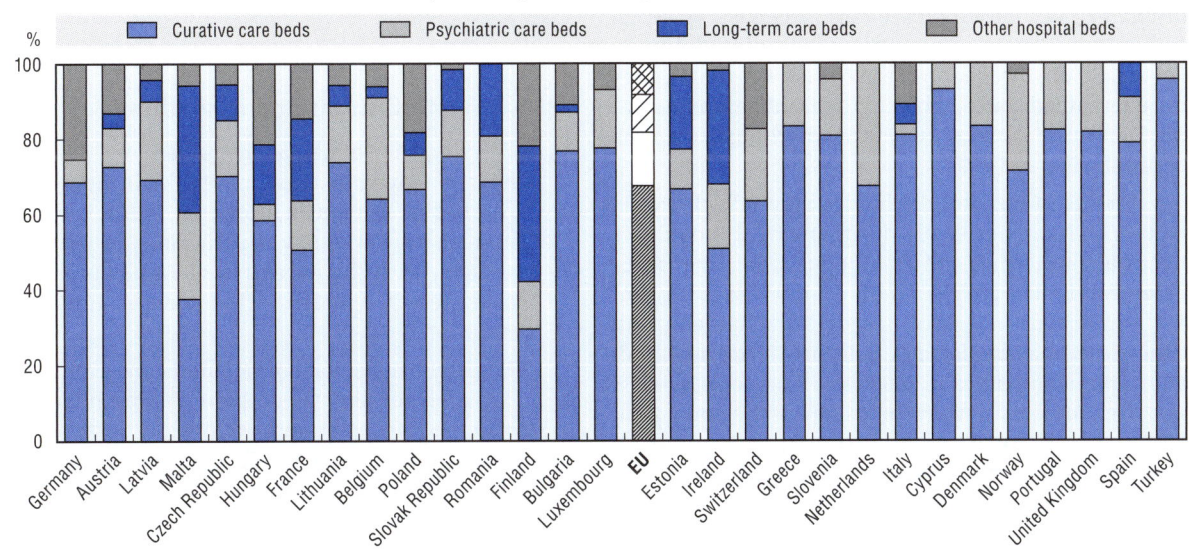

Source: OECD Health Data 2010; Eurostat Statistics Database.

StatLink http://dx.doi.org/10.1787/888932336920

Hospital discharges measure the number of people who need to stay overnight in a hospital each year. Together with the average length of stay, they are important indicators of hospital activities. Hospital activities are affected by a number of factors, including the demand for hospital services, the capacity of hospitals to treat patients, the ability of the primary care sector to prevent avoidable hospital admissions, and the availability of post-acute care settings to provide rehabilitative and long-term care services.

In 2008, hospital discharge rates were the highest in Austria and France, although the high rate in France is partly explained by the inclusion of some same-day separations (Figure 3.7.1). Discharge rates were also high in Bulgaria, Germany and Romania. They were the lowest in Cyprus, Malta and Turkey.

In general, countries that have a greater number of hospital beds also tend to have higher discharge rates. For example, the number of hospital beds per capita in Austria and Germany is more than twice than Spain and the United Kingdom, and discharge rates are also twice as large (see Indicator 3.6).

Trends in hospital discharge rates vary widely across European countries. In about one-third of EU countries (including Austria, Germany and Greece), discharge rates have increased over the past ten years. In a second group of countries (including Belgium, France, Spain, Sweden and the United Kingdom), they have remained stable, while in the third group (including Denmark, Finland and Italy), discharge rates fell between 1998 and 2008.

Trends in hospital discharges may reflect several factors that are not easily disentangled. Demand for hospitalisation may grow as populations age, since older population groups account for a disproportionately high percentage of hospital discharges in all countries. For example, in Austria and Germany, 42% of all hospital discharges in 2008 were for people aged 65 and over, more than twice their share of the population (17% and 20% respectively). However, population ageing alone may be a less important factor in explaining trends in hospitalisation rates than changes in medical technologies and clinical practices. A significant body of research shows that the diffusion of new medical interventions gradually extends to older population groups, as interventions become safer and more effective for people at older ages (e.g. Dormont and Huber, 2006). The diffusion of new medical technologies may also involve a reduction in hospitalisation if it entails a shift from procedures requiring overnight stays in hospitals to same-day procedures. In the group of countries where discharge rates have decreased over the past decade, the reduction can be explained at least partly by a strong rise in the number of day surgeries (see Indicator 3.10, for example, for evidence on the rise in day surgeries for cataracts).

Lithuania has the highest discharge rate for circulatory diseases, followed by Latvia, Bulgaria, Germany and Austria (Figure 3.7.2). The high rates in Lithuania, Latvia and Bulgaria are associated with high mortality rates from circulatory diseases, which may also be used as a proxy indicator for the occurrence of these diseases (see Indicator 1.4). This is not the case however for Germany and Austria, suggesting that different clinical practices may play a role.

Austria and Germany have the highest discharge rates for cancer, followed by Hungary (Figure 3.7.3). While the high rate in Hungary is associated with a high mortality rate from cancer (which may also be used as a proxy for the occurrence of the disease; see Indicator 1.5), this is not the case for Austria and Germany. In Austria, the high rate is associated with a high rate of hospital readmissions for further investigation and treatment of cancer patients (European Commission, 2008a).

Definition and deviations

Discharge is defined as the release of a patient who has stayed at least one night in hospital. It includes deaths in hospital following inpatient care. Same-day separations are usually excluded, with the exception of France and the Slovak Republic which include some same-day separations.

Healthy babies born in hospitals are excluded completely (or almost completely) from hospital discharge rates in several countries (e.g. Austria, Cyprus, Estonia, Finland, Greece, Ireland, Latvia, Luxembourg, Malta, Norway, Spain, Sweden, Turkey), resulting in an under-estimation of 3-6% of all discharges.

Some countries do not cover all hospitals. For instance, data for Denmark, Ireland and the United Kingdom are restricted to public or publicly-funded hospitals only. Data for Portugal relate only to public hospitals on the mainland.

3.7.1. Hospital discharges per 1 000 population, 2008 (or nearest year available)

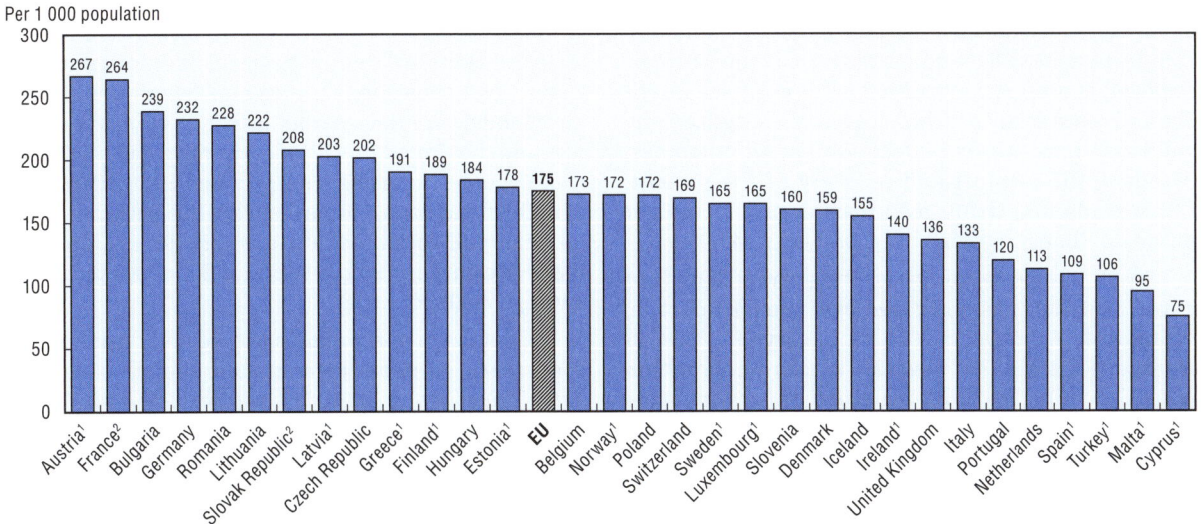

1. Excludes discharges of healthy babies born in hospital (between 3-6% of all discharges).
2. Includes same-day separations.

Source: OECD Health Data 2010; Eurostat Statistics Database.

StatLink 🔗 http://dx.doi.org/10.1787/888932336939

3.7.2. Hospital discharges for circulatory diseases per 1 000 population, 2008 (or nearest year available)

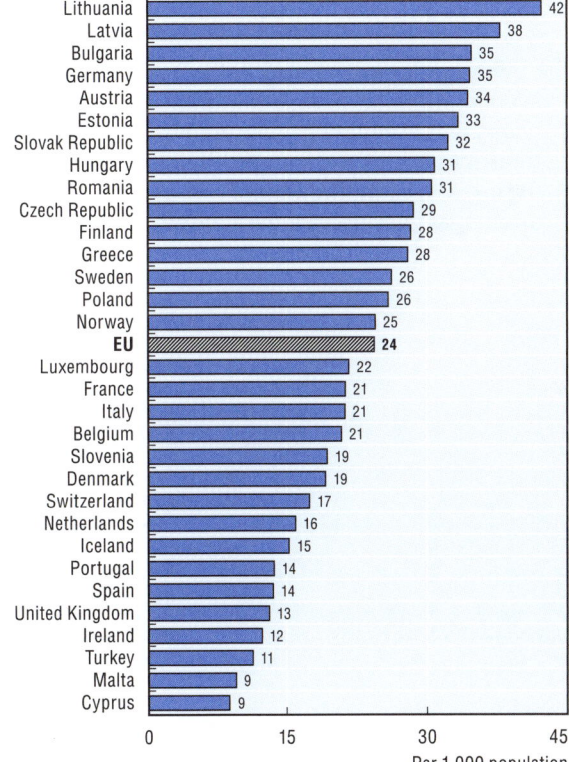

Source: OECD Health Data 2010; Eurostat Statistics Database.
StatLink 🔗 http://dx.doi.org/10.1787/888932336958

3.7.3. Hospital discharges for cancers per 1 000 population, 2008 (or nearest year available)

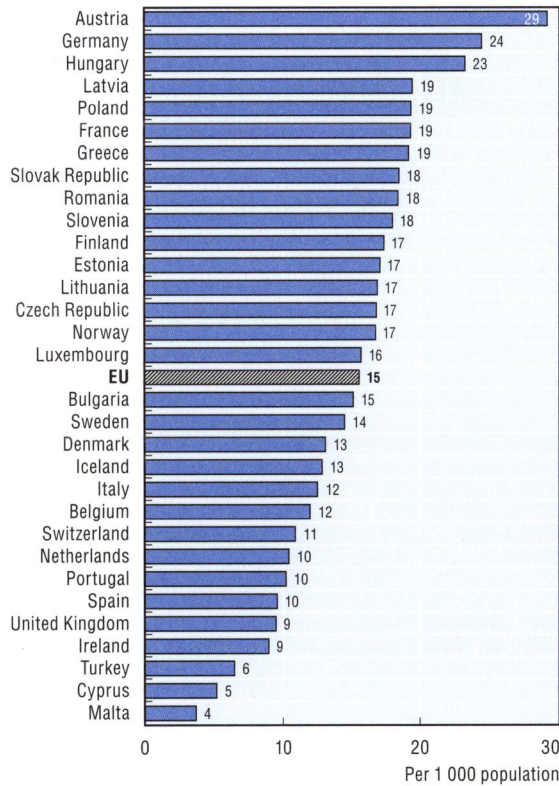

Source: OECD Health Data 2010; Eurostat Statistics Database.
StatLink 🔗 http://dx.doi.org/10.1787/888932336977

The average length of stay in hospitals is often regarded as an indicator of efficiency, since a shorter stay may reduce the cost per discharge and shift care from in-patient to less expensive post-acute settings. However, shorter stays tend to be more service intensive and more costly per day. Too short a length of stay could also have adverse effects on health outcomes, or reduce the comfort and recovery of the patient. If this leads to a rising readmission rate, costs per episode of illness may fall little, or even rise.

In all European countries, the average length of stay in hospitals has decreased over the past decade, falling from 8.3 days in 2000 to 7.2 days in 2008 on average (Figure 3.8.1). Several factors explain this general decline, including the use of less invasive surgical procedures, changes in hospital payment methods, and the expansion of early discharge programmes enabling patients to return to their home to receive follow-up care. The reduction in average length of stay was particularly marked in Switzerland (which had the highest length of stay in 2000), Bulgaria and the Netherlands. In Switzerland, the progressive move from bed-day payments to DRG-based payments has contributed to the reduction in average length of stay in those cantons that have modified their payment system (OECD and WHO, 2006).

In 2008, the average length of stay in hospitals was the lowest in Turkey, Malta, and in several Nordic countries (Norway, Denmark, Iceland, Sweden). It was the highest in Finland, followed by Switzerland and Germany. The high average length of stay in Finland is due to a large proportion of beds allocated for convalescent patients and long-term care (see Indicator 3.6). Focusing only on stays in acute care units, the average length of stay in Finland is not greater, indeed is even lower than in most other European countries.

Focusing on average length of stay for specific diseases or conditions can remove some of the heterogeneity arising from different mix and severity of conditions treated in hospitals across countries. Figure 3.8.3 shows that the average length of stay for a normal delivery ranges from less than two days in Turkey and the United Kingdom, to over five days in the Slovak Republic, Romania, Hungary and Switzerland. The length of stay for a normal delivery has become shorter in nearly all countries over the past decade, dropping from five days in 1995 to less than four days in 2008 on average in EU countries.

Lengths of stay following acute myocardial infarction (AMI, or heart attack) also declined over the past fifteen years. In 2008, it was the lowest in Turkey and some Nordic countries (Norway, Denmark and Sweden). At the other end of the scale, it was highest in Germany, Lithuania, Finland and Estonia (Figure 3.8.2). In this latter group of countries, long average length of stays may be due to the fact that some patients originally admitted for AMI are no longer receiving acute care, but nonetheless stay in hospitals for a certain period to receive post-acute care.

Definition and deviations

Average length of stay (ALOS) refers to the average number of days that patients spend in hospital. It is generally measured by dividing the total number of days stayed by all in-patients during a year by the number of admissions or discharges. Day cases are excluded.

3.8.1. Average length of stay in hospital for all causes, 2000 and 2008 (or nearest year available)

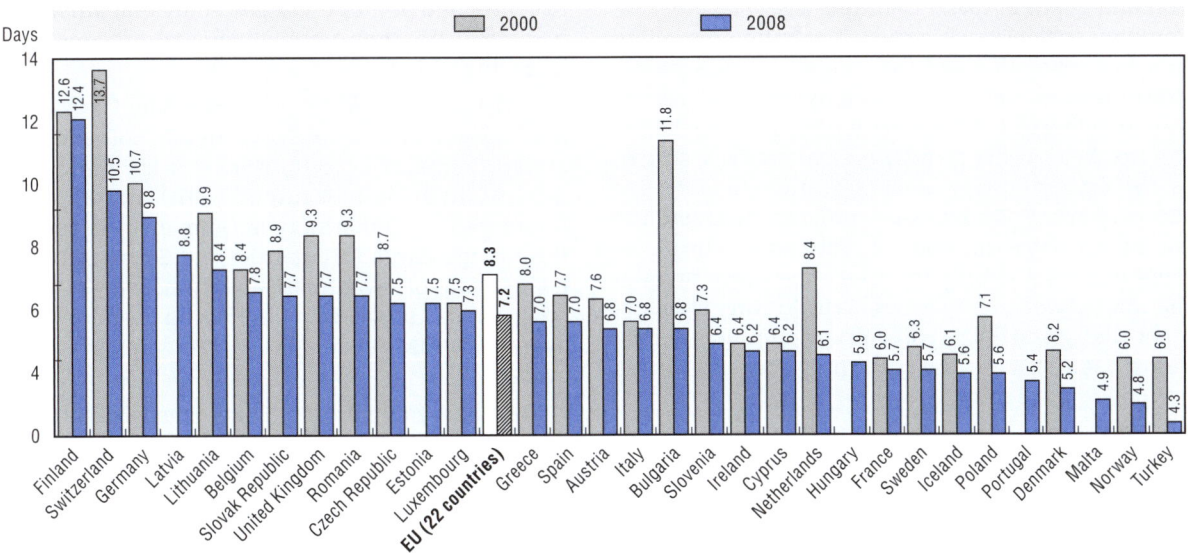

Source: OECD Health Data 2010; Eurostat Statistics Database.

StatLink ⬛ http://dx.doi.org/10.1787/888932336996

3.8.2. Average length of stay following acute myocardial infarction (AMI), 2008 (or nearest year available)

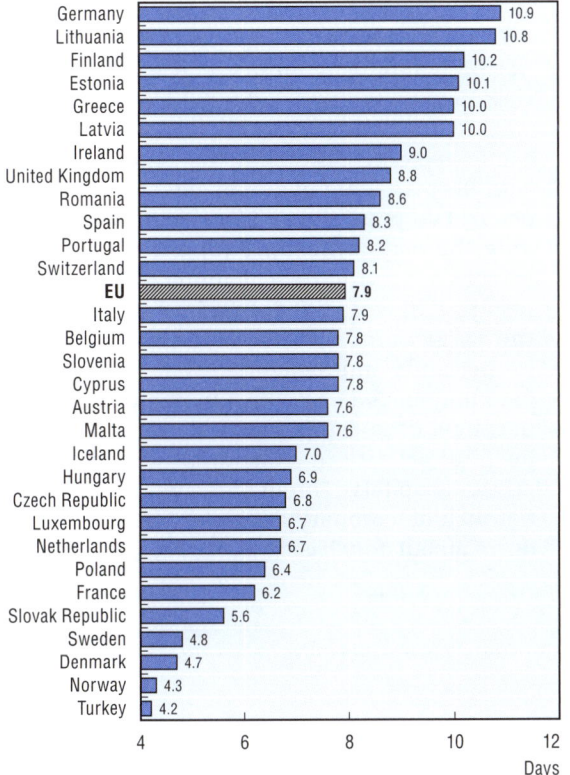

Source: OECD Health Data 2010; Eurostat Statistics Database.
StatLink ⬛ http://dx.doi.org/10.1787/888932337015

3.8.3. Average length of stay for normal delivery, 2008 (or nearest year available)

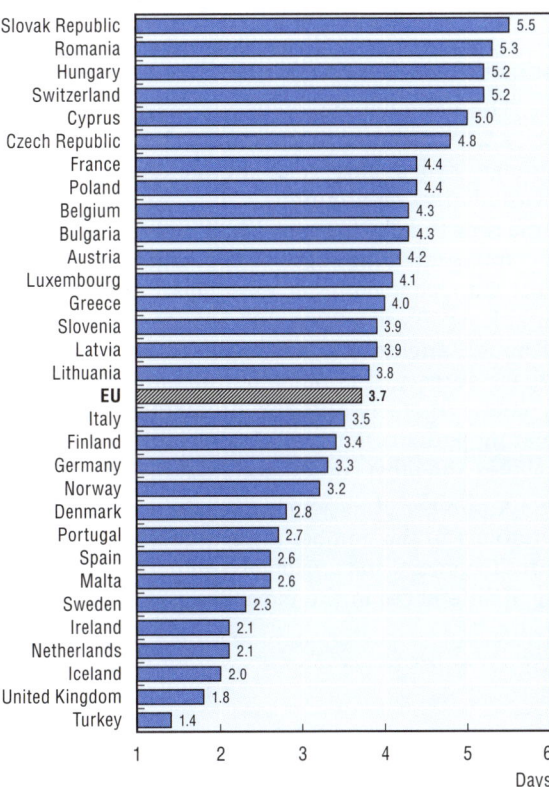

Source: OECD Health Data 2010; Eurostat Statistics Database.
StatLink ⬛ http://dx.doi.org/10.1787/888932337034

Heart diseases are a leading cause of hospitalisation and death in OECD countries (see Indicator 1.4). Coronary angioplasty is a revascularisation procedure that has revolutionised the treatment of ischemic heart diseases over the past twenty years. It involves the threading of a catheter with a balloon attached to the tip through the arterial system, usually started in the femoral artery in the leg, into the diseased coronary artery. The balloon is inflated to distend the coronary artery at the point of obstruction. The placement of a stent to keep the artery open accompanies the majority of angioplasties. Drug-eluting stents (a stent that gradually releases drugs) are increasingly being used to stem the growth of scar-like tissue surrounding the stent.

There is considerable variation across European countries in the use of coronary angioplasty (Figure 3.9.1). Germany and Belgium have the highest rates of angioplasty in 2008, followed by Italy and Norway. In Belgium, the high rate of coronary angioplasty can only be partly attributed to patient mobility. In 2006, only 2.5% of people who received an angioplasty on an in-patient basis in Belgium were non-residents (European Commission, 2008a). The rate of use of angioplasty is the lowest in the Netherlands and Switzerland, although these two countries report only the main procedure (not all procedures), resulting in a significant under-estimation (see box on definition).

The use of angioplasty has increased rapidly since 1990 in most OECD countries, overtaking coronary bypass surgery as the preferred method of revascularisation around the mid-1990s – about the same time that the first published trials of the efficacy of coronary stenting began to appear (Moïse, 2003). In most European countries, angioplasty now accounts for at least 70% of all revascularisations (Figure 3.9.2). Although angioplasty has replaced in many cases bypass surgery, it is not a perfect substitute since bypass surgery is still the preferred method for treating patients with multiple-vessel obstructions, diabetes and other conditions (Taggart, 2009).

A number of reasons can explain cross-country variations in the number of revascularisation procedures in general and angioplasty in particular, including: i) differences in the incidence and prevalence of ischemic heart diseases; ii) differences in the capacity to deliver and pay for these procedures; iii) differences in clinical treatment guidelines and practices; and iv) coding and reporting practices.

The large variations in the number of revascularisation procedures across countries do not seem to be closely related to the incidence of ischemic heart disease (IHD), as measured by IHD mortality (see Figure 1.4.1). IHD mortality in Germany is lower than the average across EU countries, but Germany has the highest rate of revascularisation procedures. On the other hand, IHD mortality in Finland is above the EU average, while revascularisation rates are below average.

Coronary angioplasty is an expensive intervention, although it is much less costly than a coronary bypass because it is less intrusive. In 2007, the average estimated price of an angioplasty was about EUR 6 000 in France, EUR 8 000 in Sweden and EUR 8 600 in Italy. Nonetheless, the estimated price of an angioplasty in Italy remains 30% lower than in the United States (Koechlin et al., 2010).

Definition and deviations

The data relate to in-patient procedures, normally counting all procedures. However, classification systems and registration practices vary across countries, and the same procedure can be recorded differently (e.g. an angioplasty with the placement of a stent can be counted as one or two procedures). Some countries report only the main procedure (or the number of patients receiving one or more procedures), resulting in a significant under-estimation of the total number. This is the case for the Netherlands and Switzerland. In Ireland, the data only include activities in publicly-funded hospitals (it is estimated that over 10% of all hospital activity in Ireland is undertaken in private hospitals). For all countries, the data do not include coronary angioplasties performed on an ambulatory basis.

3.9.1. Coronary angioplasty per 100 000 population

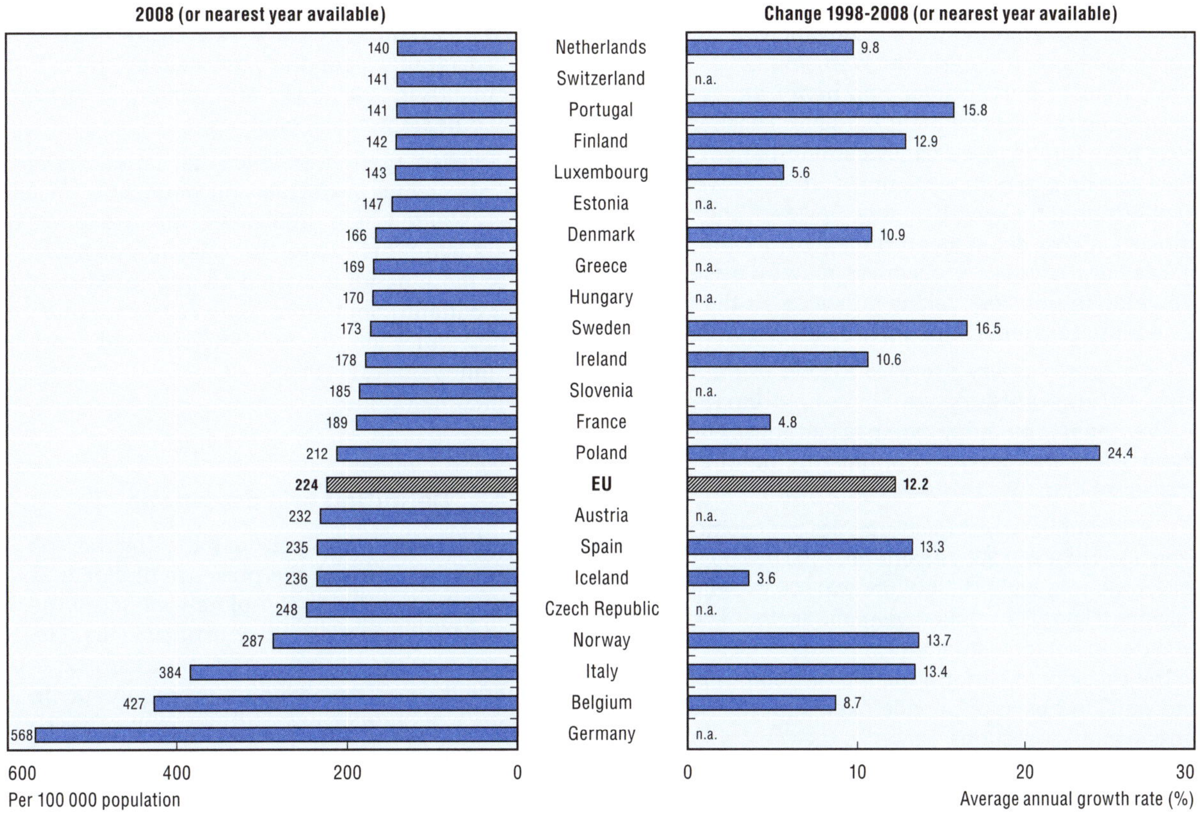

2008 (or nearest year available)		Change 1998-2008 (or nearest year available)
140	Netherlands	9.8
141	Switzerland	n.a.
141	Portugal	15.8
142	Finland	12.9
143	Luxembourg	5.6
147	Estonia	n.a.
166	Denmark	10.9
169	Greece	n.a.
170	Hungary	n.a.
173	Sweden	16.5
178	Ireland	10.6
185	Slovenia	n.a.
189	France	4.8
212	Poland	24.4
224	**EU**	**12.2**
232	Austria	n.a.
235	Spain	13.3
236	Iceland	3.6
248	Czech Republic	n.a.
287	Norway	13.7
384	Italy	13.4
427	Belgium	8.7
568	Germany	n.a.

Per 100 000 population

Average annual growth rate (%)

Note: Some of the variations across countries are due to different classification systems and recording practices.

Source: OECD Health Data 2010.

StatLink ᴍᴤᴸ *http://dx.doi.org/10.1787/888932337053*

3.9.2. Coronary angioplasty as a percentage of total revascularisation procedures, 1998-2008

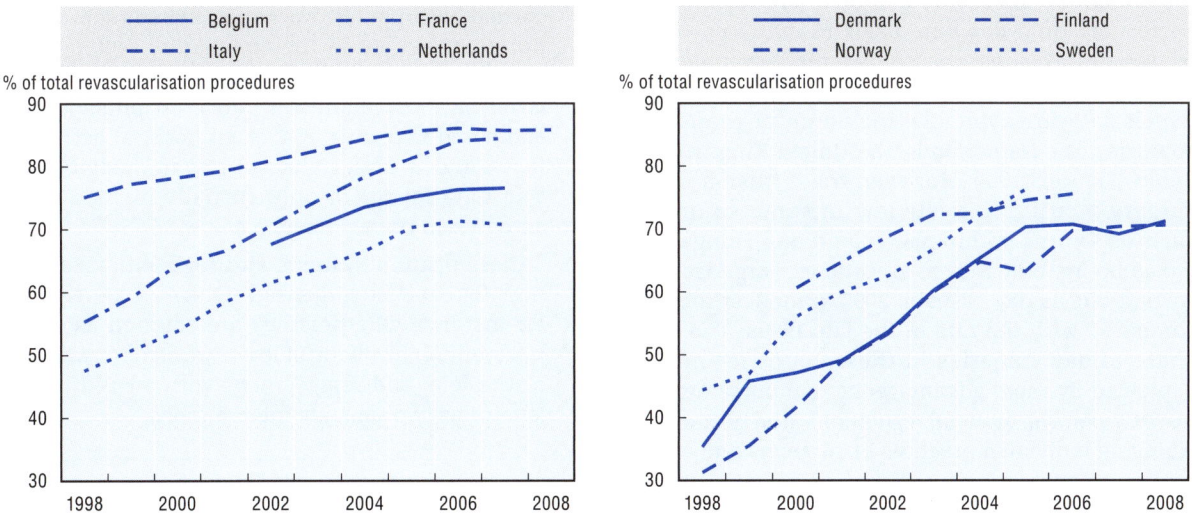

Legend (left chart): Belgium — France — - - - Italy — · — · Netherlands · · · · · ·

Legend (right chart): Denmark — Finland — - - - Norway — · — · Sweden · · · · · ·

Note: Revascularisation procedures include coronary bypass and angioplasty.

Source: OECD Health Data 2010.

StatLink ᴍᴤᴸ *http://dx.doi.org/10.1787/888932337072*

In the past 20 years, the number of surgical procedures carried out on a day care basis has steadily grown in European countries. Advances in medical technologies, particularly the diffusion of less invasive surgical interventions, and better anaesthetics have made this development possible. These innovations have improved effectiveness and patient safety. They also help to reduce the unit cost of interventions by shortening the length of stay. However, the overall impact on cost depends on the extent to which any greater use of these procedures may be offset by a reduction in unit cost, taking into account the cost of post-acute care and community health services.

Cataract surgery provides a good example of a high volume surgery which is now carried out predominantly on a day care basis in most European countries. It has become the most frequent surgical procedure in many European countries.

The number of cataract surgeries per capita ranges from a low of about 200 surgeries per 100 000 population in Cyprus to a high of 1 848 per 100 000 population in Belgium (Figure 3.10.1). Both demand factors (including an older population structure) and supply factors (such as the capacity to perform the intervention in hospital and outside hospital) provide explanations for these cross-country variations. However, the comparability of data is also limited by registration procedures, particularly the lack of registration of day surgeries carried outside hospitals in some countries, which explain the low rates in Ireland, Poland and Denmark. The very high rate in countries such as Belgium may be explained partly by the registration of more than one procedure per surgery.

Cataract surgeries are now predominantly performed on a day care basis in many European countries. Day surgery accounts for 90% or more of all cataract surgeries in about half of the countries for which data are available, including in the Nordic countries, the Netherlands, the United Kingdom and Spain (Figure 3.10.2). However, the diffusion of day surgery is still relatively low in some countries, such as Cyprus, Lithuania, Poland and Hungary. In Luxembourg, only 35% of all cataract surgeries were carried out as day cases in 2007, a modest increase compared with the rate in the late 1990s. The small share of day surgeries in these countries may be explained by more advantageous reimbursement for in-patient stays, national regulations, and obstacles to changing individual practices of surgeons and anaesthetists (Castoro et al., 2007), together with limitations in data coverage. In France, the share of cataract surgeries carried out on a same-day basis has increased rapidly over the past decade, from 23% in 1998 to 70% in 2007, but it still remains below that of many other European countries.

In Sweden, there is evidence that cataract surgeries are now being performed on patients suffering from less severe vision problems compared to five or ten years ago. This raises the question of how the needs of these patients should be prioritised relative to other patient populations (Swedish Association of Local Authorities and Regions and National Board of Health and Welfare, 2008).

Definition and deviations

Cataract surgeries consist of removing the lens of the eye because of the presence of cataracts which are partially or completely clouding the lens, and replacing it with an artificial lens. The surgery may be carried out as day cases or as in-patient cases (involving an overnight stay in hospital). Same-day interventions may either be performed in a hospital or in a clinic. However, the data for many countries (e.g. Ireland, Hungary, Poland) only include interventions carried out in hospitals. Caution is therefore required in making cross-country comparisons of available data, given the incomplete coverage of day surgeries in several countries.

Denmark only includes cataract surgeries carried out in public hospitals, excluding procedures carried out in the ambulatory sector and in private hospitals. In Ireland too, the data cover only procedures in public hospitals (it is estimated that over 10% of all hospital activity in Ireland is undertaken in private hospitals). The data for Spain only partially include the activities in private hospitals.

Classification systems and registration practices for cataract surgeries vary across countries, for instance whether they are counted as one intervention involving at least two steps (removal or the lens and replacement with an artificial lens) or as two separate interventions.

3.10.1. Number of cataract surgeries, in-patient and day cases, per 100 000 population, 1998 and 2008 (or nearest year available)

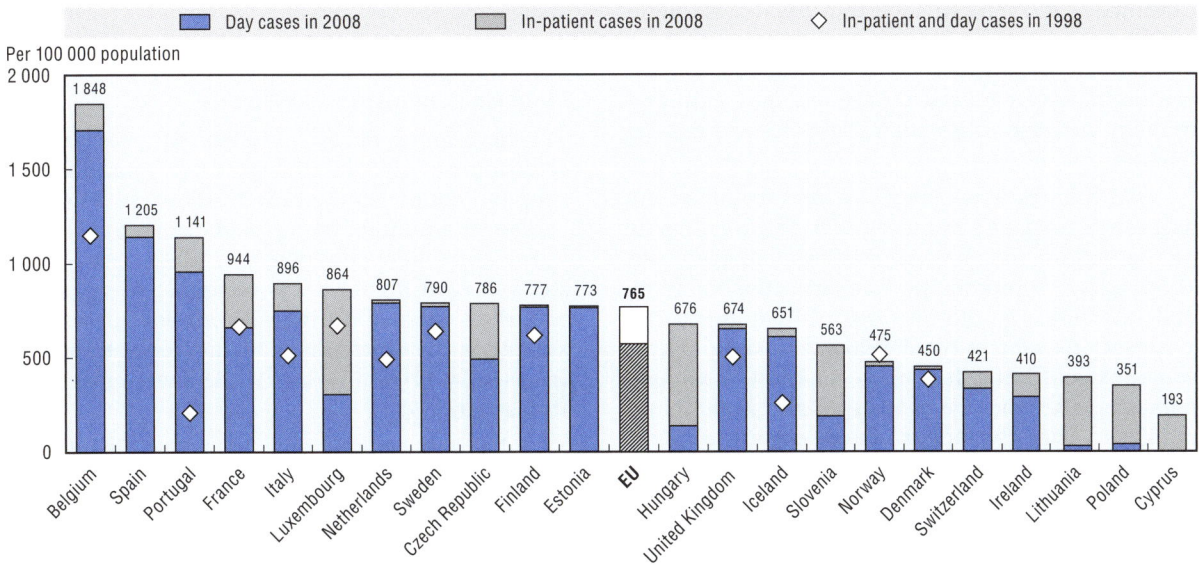

Note: Some of the variations across countries are due to different classification systems and recording practices.

Source: OECD Health Data 2010; Eurostat Statistics Database.

StatLink http://dx.doi.org/10.1787/888932337091

3.10.2. Share of cataract surgeries carried out as day cases, 1998 and 2008 (or nearest year available)

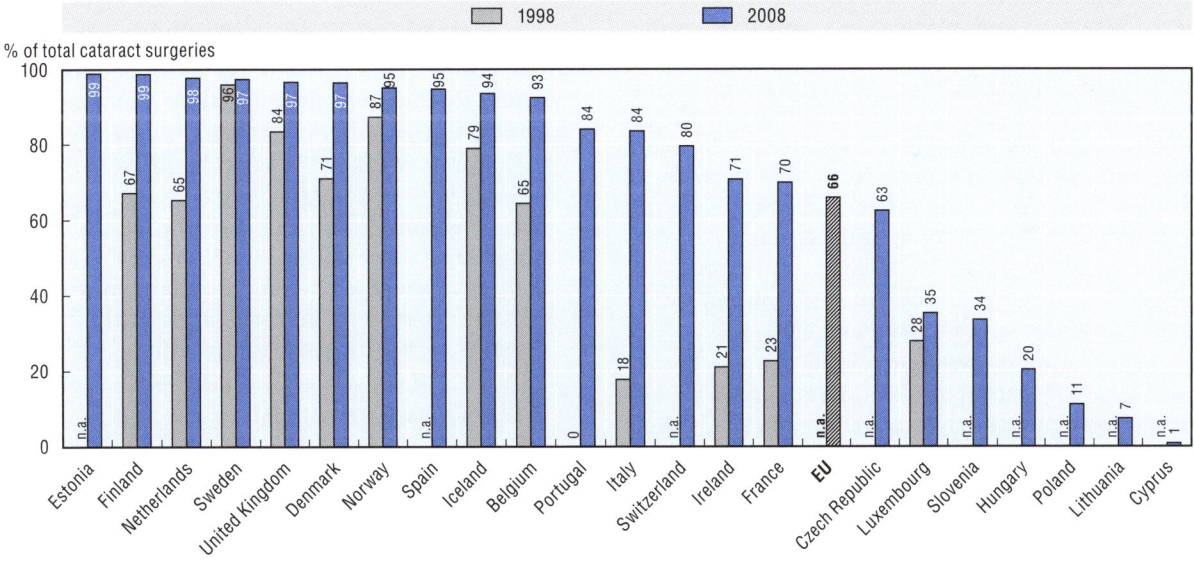

Source: OECD Health Data 2010; Eurostat Statistics Database.

StatLink http://dx.doi.org/10.1787/888932337110

Significant advancements in surgical treatment have provided effective options to reduce the pain and disability associated with certain musculoskeletal conditions. Joint replacement surgery (hip and knee replacement) is considered the most effective intervention for severe osteoarthritis, reducing pain and disability and restoring some patients to near normal function.

Ostheoarthritis is one of the ten most disabling diseases in developed countries. Worldwide estimates are that 9.6% of men and 18.0% of women aged over 60 years have symptomatic osteoarthritis, including moderate and severe forms (WHO, 2010a). Age is the strongest predictor of the development and progression of osteoarthritis. It is more common in women, increasing after the age of 50 especially in the hand and knee. Other risk factors include obesity, physical inactivity, smoking, excess alcohol and injuries (European Commission, 2008b). While joint replacement surgery is mainly carried out among people aged 60 and over, it can also be performed among people at younger ages.

There is considerable variation across countries in the rate of hip and knee replacement (Figures 3.11.1 and 3.11.2). Germany, Austria, Belgium, Norway and Switzerland have the highest rates of hip replacement. These countries are also amongst those that have the highest rates of knee replacement. A number of reasons can explain these cross-country variations in the rate of hip and knee replacement, including: i) differences in the prevalence of osteoarthritis problems; ii) differences in the capacity to deliver and pay for these expensive procedures; iii) differences in clinical treatment guidelines and practices; and iv) international mobility of patients across borders (e.g. in Belgium, about 2% of knee replacement are performed on people who are not residing in the country; European Commission, 2008a).

There are too few comparable studies on the prevalence of osteoarthritis in Europe to draw any conclusions on cross-country variations. Nor is there any evidence as to whether the age- and sex-specific incidence of osteoarthritis has changed in recent decades. However, the number of people suffering from osteoarthritis has increased, and is expected to continue to increase in the coming years, for two reasons: 1) population ageing, which is resulting in a growing number of people over 60 and 65 years with a greater risk of suffering from osteoarthritis (even if the age and sex specific rate does not increase); and 2) the growing prevalence of obesity, which is the main risk factor for osteoarthritis beyond age and sex (European Commission, 2008b).

The number of hip and knee replacement has increased rapidly over the past ten years in most European countries (Figures 3.11.3 and 3.11.4). On average, the number of hip replacement increased by one-third between 1998 and 2008. The growth rate was even higher for knee replacement, which more than doubled during this ten-year period. For example, in the United Kingdom, hip replacement rate increased by 40% since 2000, while knee replacement increased by 112%.

A hip or knee replacement is an expensive intervention, although the cost varies across countries. In 2007, the average estimated price of a knee replacement in France was EUR 10 600, about 20-25% more than in Finland, Germany, Portugal and Sweden. Nonetheless, the estimated price of a knee replacement in France remained 15-20% lower than in the United States (Koechlin *et al.*, 2010).

Definition and deviations

Hip replacement is a surgical procedure in which the hip joint is replaced by a prosthetic implant. It is generally conducted to relieve arthritis pain or treat severe physical joint damage following hip fracture.

Knee replacement is a surgical procedure to replace the weight-bearing surfaces of the knee joint to relieve the pain and disability of osteoarthritis. It may be performed for other knee diseases such as rheumatoid arthritis.

Classification systems and registration practices vary across countries, which may affect the comparability of the data. In Ireland, the data only include activities in publicly-funded hospitals (it is estimated that over 10% of all hospital activity in Ireland is undertaken in private hospitals).

3.11.1. Hip replacement surgery, per 100 000 population, 2008 (or nearest year available)

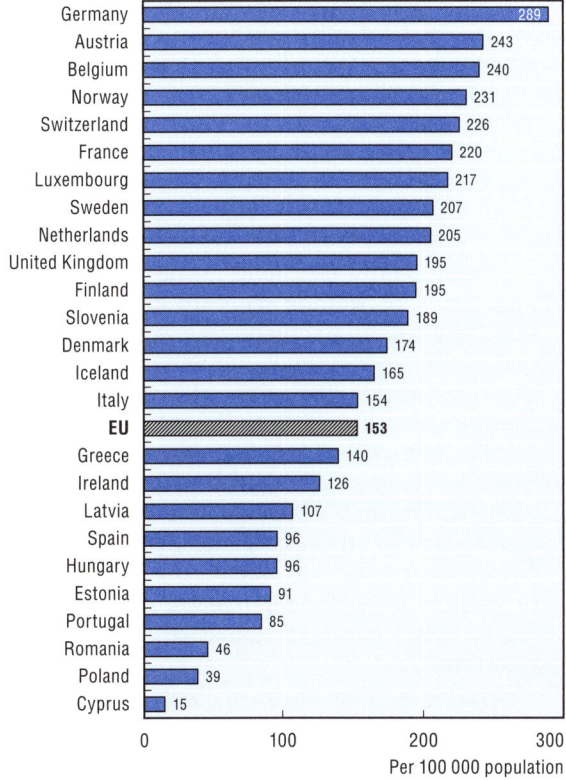

Source: OECD Health Data 2010; Eurostat Statistics Database.
StatLink http://dx.doi.org/10.1787/888932337129

3.11.3. Trend in hip replacement surgery, 1998 to 2008 (or nearest year available), selected countries

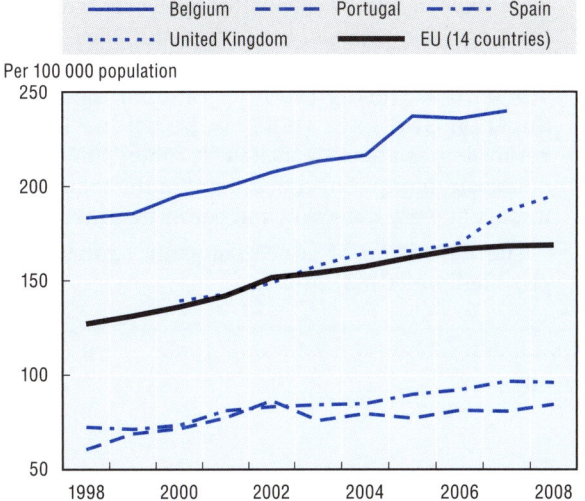

Source: OECD Health Data 2010; Eurostat Statistics Database.
StatLink http://dx.doi.org/10.1787/888932337167

3.11.2. Knee replacement surgery, per 100 000 population, 2008 (or nearest year available)

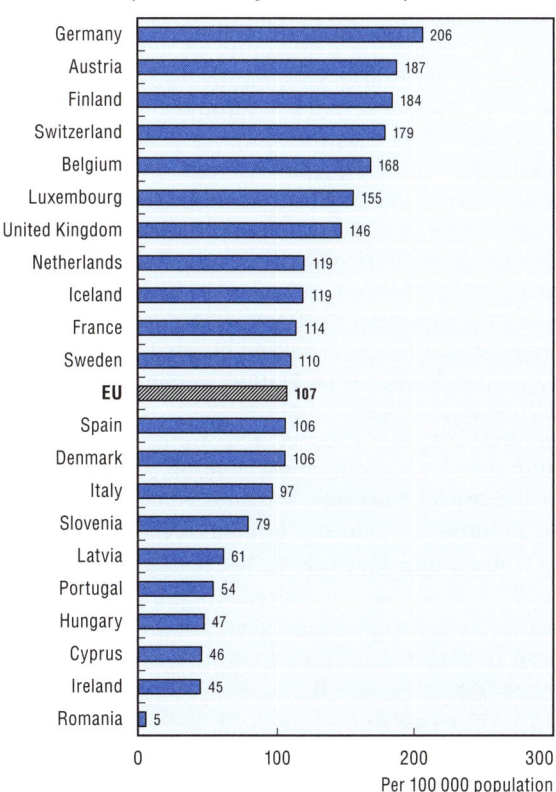

Source: OECD Health Data 2010; Eurostat Statistics Database.
StatLink http://dx.doi.org/10.1787/888932337148

3.11.4. Trend in knee replacement surgery, 1998 to 2008 (or nearest year available), selected countries

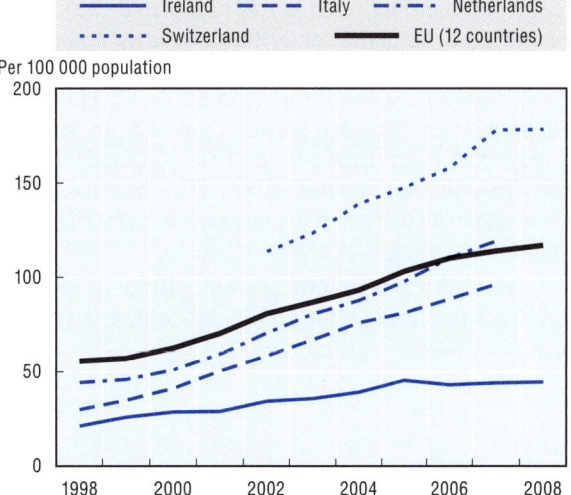

Source: OECD Health Data 2010; Eurostat Statistics Database.
StatLink http://dx.doi.org/10.1787/888932337186

Cervical cancer is largely preventable. Screening by regular pelvic exam and pap smears can identify premalignant lesions, which can be effectively treated before the occurrence of the cancer. Regular screening also increases the probability of diagnosing early stages of the cancer and improving survival. Consequently, the Council of the European Union and the European Commission promote population based cancer screening programmes among member states (European Union, 2003; European Commission, 2008c) and European countries have instituted screening programmes with specific periodicity and target groups. In addition, promising cancer preventing vaccines have been developed based on the discovery that cervical cancer is caused by sexual transmission of certain forms of the Human Papilloma Virus. The efficacy and safety of those vaccines is now well established, but debates about cost-effectiveness and the implications of vaccination programmes for teenagers for a sexually transmitted disease continue in a number of countries (Huang, 2008).

Screening rates vary widely across countries with Austria, Norway, the United Kingdom and Sweden achieving coverage of around 80% of the target population (Figure 3.12.1). Some countries with very low screening rates, like Turkey and Latvia, did not have uniform national screening programme as of 2008; the low rates reflect local programmes or opportunistic screening. Screening rates in several countries declined slightly between 2000 and 2008.

Relative survival rates are commonly used to track progress in treating cancer over time as they reflect both how early the cancer was detected and the effectiveness of the treatment provided. Survival rates have been used to compare European countries in the EUROCARE study, in comparisons between European countries and the United States (Gatta et al., 2000), and in national reporting activities in many countries. Nearly all countries recorded five-year relative survival rates above 60% for the period 2002-07. The rates ranged from 71% in Iceland to 50% in Poland (Figure 3.12.2). Over the periods 1997-2002 and 2002-07, the five-year relative rates improved in most countries, although in all instances the increase is not statistically significant.

Mortality rates alone are not sufficient to draw timely inferences about quality of care, but current cancer mortality rates reflect the effect of care in past years and changes in incidence. Mortality rates for cervical cancer are higher in eastern European countries (Figure 3.12.3). Between 1998 and 2008 the rates declined for most European countries, with larger improvements for Iceland, Denmark, Slovenia, the Czech Republic and Norway.

Definitions and deviations

Screening rates for cervical cancer reflect the proportion of women who are eligible for a screening test and actually receive the test. As policies regarding screening periodicity differ across countries, the rates are based on each country's specific policy. An important consideration is that some countries ascertain screening based on surveys and other based on encounter data, which may influence the results. If a country has an organised screening programme, but women receive care outside the programme, rates may be underreported. Survey-based results may also underestimate the rates due to recall bias.

Relative cancer survival rates reflect the proportion of patients with a certain type of cancer who are still alive after a specified time period (commonly five years) compared to those still alive in absence of the disease. Relative survival rates capture the excess mortality that can be attributed to the diagnosis. For example, a relative survival rate of 80% does not mean that 80% of the cancer patients are still alive after five years, but that 80% of the patients that were expected to be alive after five years, given their age at diagnosis, are in fact still alive. All the survival rates presented here have been age-standardised using the International Cancer Survival Standard (ICSS) population. The survival rates are not adjusted for tumor stage at diagnosis, hampering assessment of the relative impact of early detection and better treatment.

The definition of cancer mortality rates is provided under Indicator 1.5.

3.12.1. Cervical cancer screening, percentage of women screened aged 20-69, 2000 to 2008 (or nearest year)

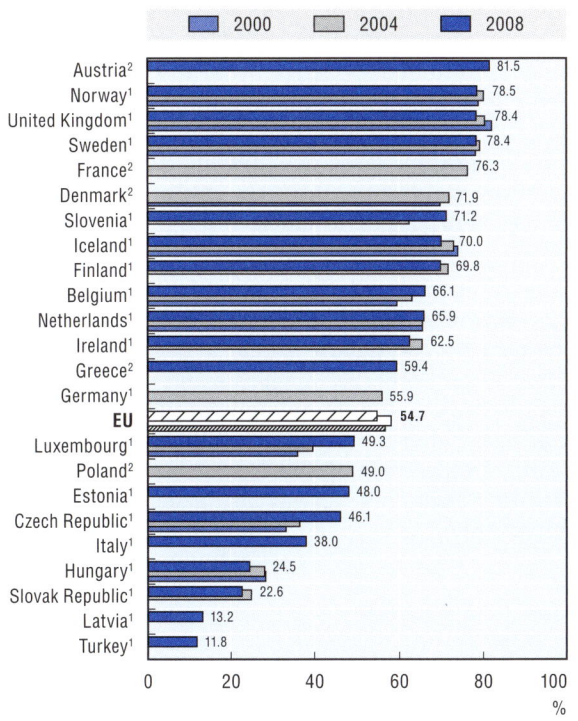

Legend: 2000, 2004, 2008

	%
Austria[2]	81.5
Norway[1]	78.5
United Kingdom[1]	78.4
Sweden[1]	78.4
France[2]	76.3
Denmark[2]	71.9
Slovenia[1]	71.2
Iceland[1]	70.0
Finland[1]	69.8
Belgium[1]	66.1
Netherlands[1]	65.9
Ireland[1]	62.5
Greece[2]	59.4
Germany[1]	55.9
EU	**54.7**
Luxembourg[1]	49.3
Poland[2]	49.0
Estonia[1]	48.0
Czech Republic[1]	46.1
Italy[1]	38.0
Hungary[1]	24.5
Slovak Republic[1]	22.6
Latvia[1]	13.2
Turkey[1]	11.8

1. Programme.
2. Survey.
Source: OECD Health Data 2010.

StatLink http://dx.doi.org/10.1787/888932337205

3.12.2. Cervical cancer five-year relative survival rate, 1997-2002 and 2002-07 (or nearest period)

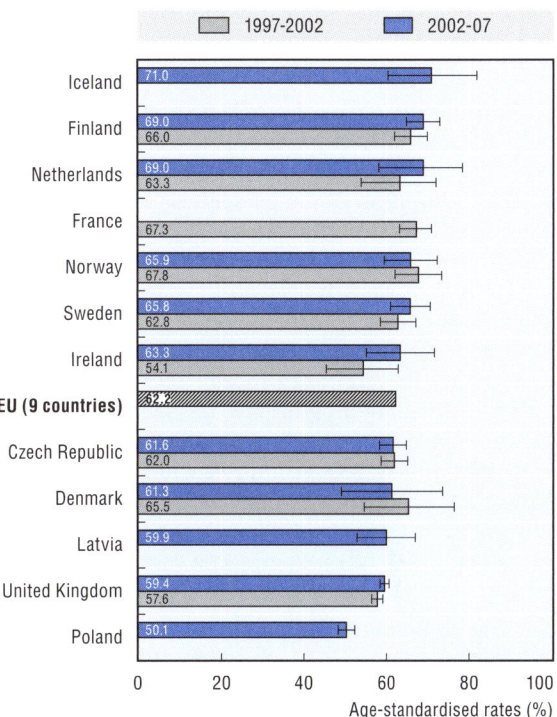

Legend: 1997-2002, 2002-07

	Age-standardised rates (%)
Iceland	71.0
Finland	69.0 / 66.0
Netherlands	69.0 / 63.3
France	67.3
Norway	65.9 / 67.8
Sweden	65.8 / 62.8
Ireland	63.3 / 54.1
EU (9 countries)	**62.2**
Czech Republic	61.6 / 62.0
Denmark	61.3 / 65.5
Latvia	59.9
United Kingdom	59.4 / 57.6
Poland	50.1

Source: OECD Health Care Quality Indicators Data 2009 (survival rates are age-standardised to the International Cancer Survival Standards population and 95% confidence intervals are represented by ⊢).

StatLink http://dx.doi.org/10.1787/888932337224

3.12.3. Cervical cancer mortality, females, 1998 to 2008 (or nearest year available)

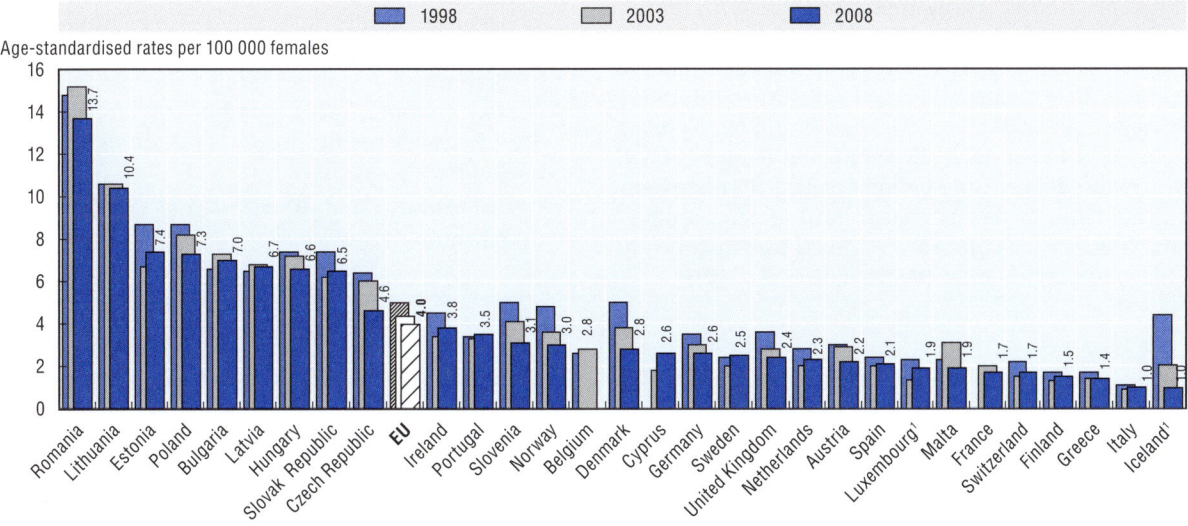

Legend: 1998, 2003, 2008

Age-standardised rates per 100 000 females

Romania 13.7, Lithuania 10.4, Estonia 7.4, Poland 7.3, Bulgaria 7.0, Latvia 6.7, Hungary 6.6, Slovak Republic 6.5, Czech Republic 4.6, EU 4.0, Ireland 3.8, Portugal 3.5, Slovenia 3.1, Norway 3.0, Belgium 2.8, Denmark 2.8, Cyprus 2.6, Germany 2.6, Sweden 2.5, United Kingdom 2.4, Netherlands 2.3, Austria 2.2, Spain 2.1, Luxembourg[1] 1.9, Malta 1.9, France 1.7, Switzerland 1.7, Finland 1.5, Greece 1.4, Italy 1.0, Iceland[1]

1. Rates for Iceland and Luxembourg are based on a three-year average to reduce year-to-year variation due to small numbers.
Source: Eurostat Statistics Database (mortality data are age-standardised to the WHO European standard population).

StatLink http://dx.doi.org/10.1787/888932337243

Breast cancer is the most common form of cancer among women in all EU countries, accounting for 31% of cancer incidence, and 17% of cancer deaths among women in 2008 (see Indicator 1.5). Overall spending for breast cancer care typically amounts to about 0.5-0.6% of total health care expenditure (OECD, 2003).

Most countries have adopted screening programmes, although the optimal frequency of screening and the target age-group are still the subject of debate. European Union guidelines (2006) promote a target screening rate of at least 75% of eligible women in European countries. In Finland and the Netherlands, close to 85% of women aged 50-69 years are screened, but rates are below 20% in Turkey, Poland, the Slovak Republic, and Denmark (Figure 3.13.1). In some countries with low screening rates, like Denmark, no national screening programme has been put in place yet; the low rates reflect opportunistic screening or local programmes. Some countries which had low rates in the early 2000s, such as the Czech Republic, showed substantial increases by 2008, whereas some countries with already high rates experienced declines, including Norway, Finland and the United Kingdom.

The combination of public health interventions and improved medical technology has contributed to substantial improvements in survival rates for breast cancer. Greater awareness of the disease and the promotion of self-examination and screening mammography (European Union, 2003; European Commission, 2006) have led to the detection of the disease at earlier stages. In addition, clinical studies have demonstrated that technological improvements, such as the introduction of combined breast conserving surgery with radiation therapy and routine adjuvant chemotherapy treatment, have increased survival as well as the quality of life of survivors (Mauri et al., 2008). Across European countries, relative five-year breast cancer survival rates have improved between 1997-2002 and 2002-07, even though changes are usually not statistically significant (Figure 3.13.2). Data over a longer time period confirm that five-year survival rates for breast cancer have increased particularly in eastern European countries that historically had lower survival rates (Verdecchia et al., 2007).

Many OECD countries have attained survival rates of over 80%, with rates as high as 88% for Iceland (Figure 3.13.2). Finland and the Netherlands, two countries that had among the highest screening rates in 2000, also report high survival rates for women diagnosed in 2002-07. Given that the effect of early detection through screening requires several years before it is manifested, the impact of the decrease in mammography rates over recent years in several countries will remain uncertain until survival rates for future years become available.

While there has been an increase in incidence rates of breast cancer in many European countries, mortality rates have declined or remained stable over the past decade (Figure 3.13.3), reflecting increased survival due to earlier diagnosis and/or better treatments. Improvements are substantial for countries that had higher mortality levels in the 1990s such as Malta, Denmark and the Netherlands, but other countries including Norway also experienced a large improvement.

Definitions and deviations

Mammography screening rates reflect the proportion of eligible women patients who are actually screened. As policies regarding target age groups and screening periodicity differ across countries, the rates are based on each country's specific policy. Some countries ascertain screening based on surveys and others based on encounter data, and this may influence results. If a country has an organised screening programme, but women receive care outside of the programme, rates may be underreported. Survey-based results may also underestimate rates due to recall bias.

Survival rates and mortality rates are defined in Indicator 3.12.

3.13.1. Mammography screening, percentage of women aged 50-69 screened, 2000 to 2008 (or nearest year)

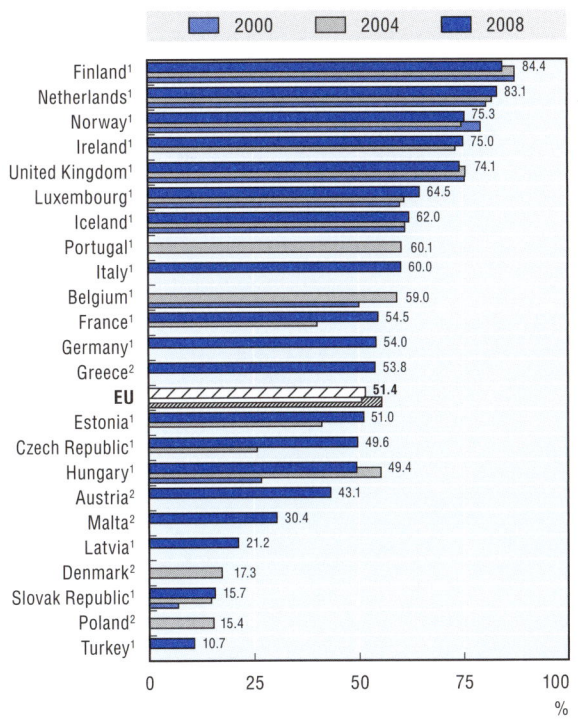

3.13.2. Breast cancer five-year relative survival rate, 1997-2002 and 2002-07 (or nearest period)

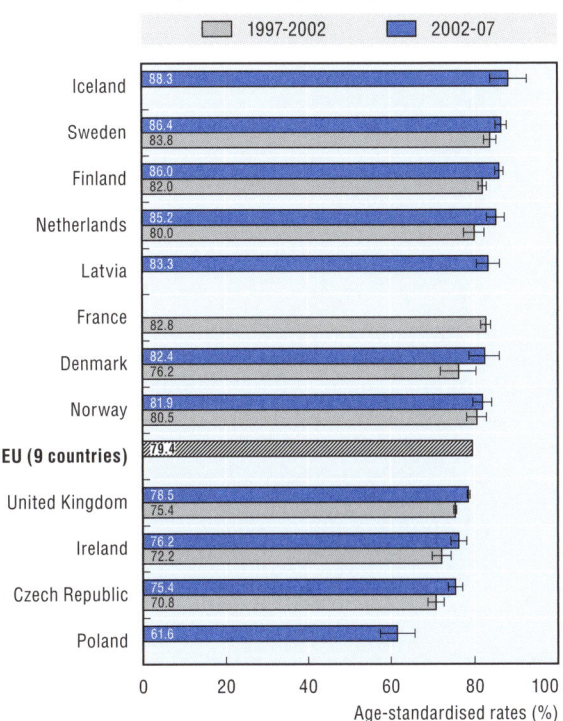

1. Programme.
2. Survey.
Source: OECD Health Data 2010.

StatLink ⬛️ http://dx.doi.org/10.1787/888932337262

Source: OECD Health Care Quality Indicators Data 2009 (survival rates are age-standardised to the International Cancer Survival Standards population and 95% confidence intervals are represented by ⊢).

StatLink ⬛️ http://dx.doi.org/10.1787/888932337281

3.13.3. Breast cancer mortality, females, 1998 to 2008 (or nearest year available)

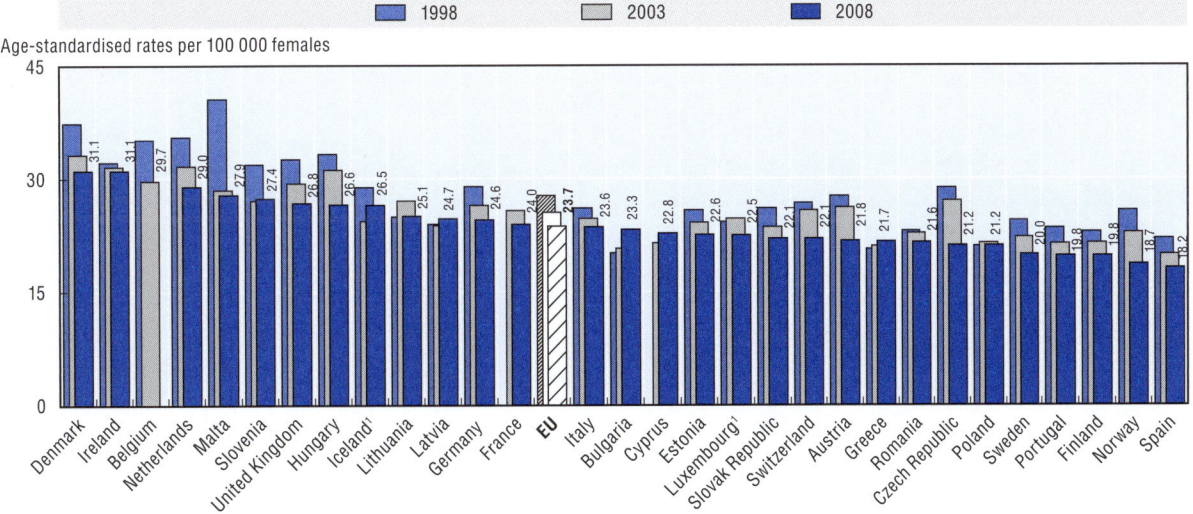

1. Rates for Iceland and Luxembourg are based on a three-year average to reduce year-to-year variation due to small numbers.

Source: Eurostat Statistics Database (mortality data are age-standardised to the WHO European standard population).

StatLink ⬛️ http://dx.doi.org/10.1787/888932337300

Chapter 4

Health Expenditure and Financing

In 2008, Norway recorded the highest spending per person on health goods and services among European countries at about EUR 4 300 (Figure 4.1.1) – almost twice the average of European Union countries. This was nonetheless far below the health spending per capita in the United States. Switzerland, Luxembourg and Austria were the next highest spending countries in Europe. Most northern and western European countries spent between EUR PPP 2 500 and 3 500 per person, that is, between 10% and 60% more than the EU average. Those countries spending below the EU average are eastern and southern European countries such as Turkey, Romania, Bulgaria, Poland and Hungary.

Figure 4.1.1 shows the breakdown of per capita spending on health into public and private components (see also Indicator 4.5). Both the ranking and the variation in the levels of public spending on health is similar to that observed for total spending on health.

Over the past ten years (1998-2008) per capita health spending is estimated to have grown in real terms by 4.6% annually on average across the EU countries (Figure 4.1.2). In many countries, the growth rate reached a peak around 2001-02 and has slowed in more recent years.

In general, the countries that have experienced the highest growth in health spending over this period are those that had relatively low levels at the beginning of the period. Health expenditure per capita growth in Turkey, for example, has generally been more than twice the EU average over the past ten years. Other countries, such as Ireland and the United Kingdom, pursued specific policy objectives to increase public spending on health, meaning that overall health spending has outpaced economic growth (Department of Health and Children, 2001; Secretary of State for Health, 2002).

In contrast, health spending per capita in Germany increased in real terms by only 1.8% per year on average over the past decade, reflecting the effect of cost-containment policies. These measures have included budget or spending caps for sectors or individual providers, promoting the use of generic drugs, restricting the number of hospital beds and high cost medical equipment, and introducing or increasing co-payments for certain services (Busse and Riesberg, 2004).

Health spending per capita in Norway in *nominal terms* grew at a fairly strong rate of nearly 7% per year over the past ten years. However, when deflated by the economy-wide price index, growth in *real terms* was relatively low (0.8%). This is because the economy-wide price index in Norway is heavily influenced by the price of oil which increased rapidly during that period.

Figure 4.1.3 shows the positive association between GDP per capita and health expenditure per capita across European countries. While there is an overall tendency for countries with higher GDP to spend a greater amount on health, there is wide variation since GDP is not the sole factor influencing health expenditure levels. The association is stronger among European countries with low GDP per capita than among countries with a higher GDP per capita. Even for countries with similar levels of GDP per capita there are substantial differences in health expenditure. For example, Spain and France have similar GDP per capita, but Spain spends less than 80% of the level of France on health.

Definition and deviations

Total expenditure on health measures the final consumption of health goods and services (i.e. current health expenditure) plus capital investment in health care infrastructure, as defined in the System of Health Accounts manual (OECD, 2000). This includes spending by both public and private sources on medical services and goods, public health and prevention programmes, and administration.

The vast majority of countries now produce health spending data according to the boundaries and definitions proposed in the System of Health Accounts manual. The comparability of the functional breakdown of health expenditure data has improved over recent years. However, limitations remain, as some countries have not yet implemented the SHA classifications and definitions. Even among those countries that are submitting data according to the SHA, the comparability of data sometimes needs to be improved. Different practices regarding the inclusion of long-term care in health or social expenditure are also a factor affecting data comparability.

Countries' health expenditures are converted to a common currency (Euro) and are adjusted to take account of the different purchasing power of the national currencies, in order to compare spending levels. Economy-wide (GDP) PPPs are used as the most available and reliable conversion rates.

4.1.1. Total health expenditure per capita, public and private, 2008

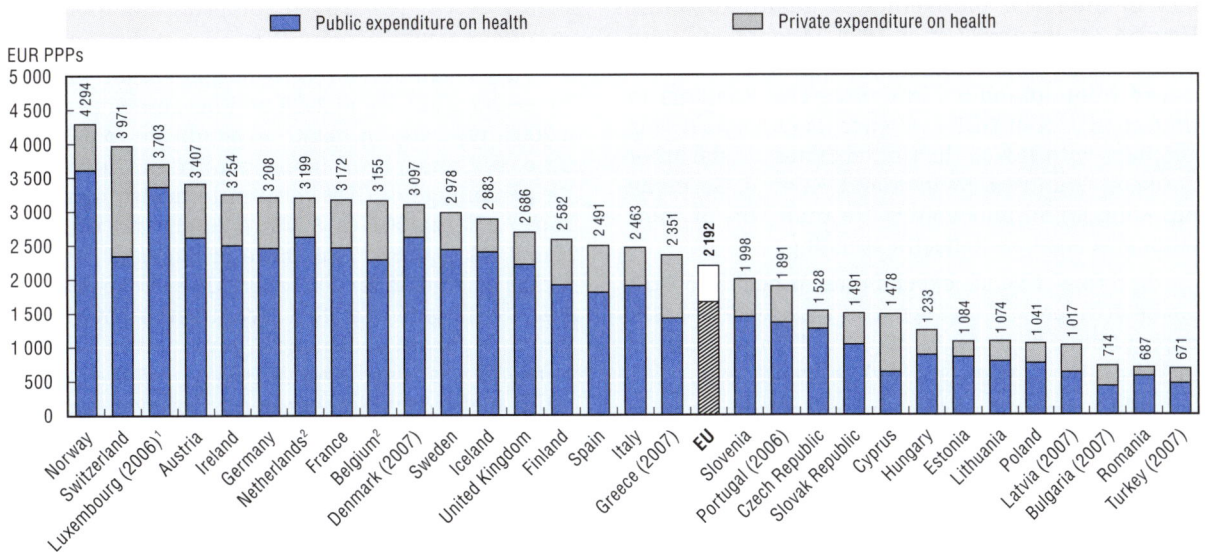

1. Health expenditure is for the insured population rather than resident population.
2. Current health expenditure (excluding investment).

Source: OECD Health Data 2010; Eurostat Statistics Database.

StatLink 🔗 *http://dx.doi.org/10.1787/888932337319*

4.1.2. Annual average growth rate in real health expenditure per capita, 1998-2008

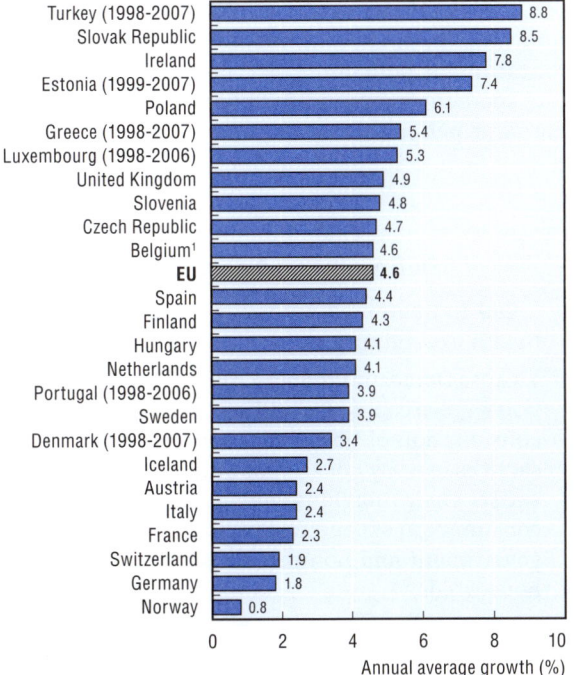

1. Current health expenditure (excluding investment).
Source: OECD Health Data 2010; Eurostat Statistics Database.

StatLink 🔗 *http://dx.doi.org/10.1787/888932337338*

4.1.3. Total health expenditure per capita and GDP per capita, 2008

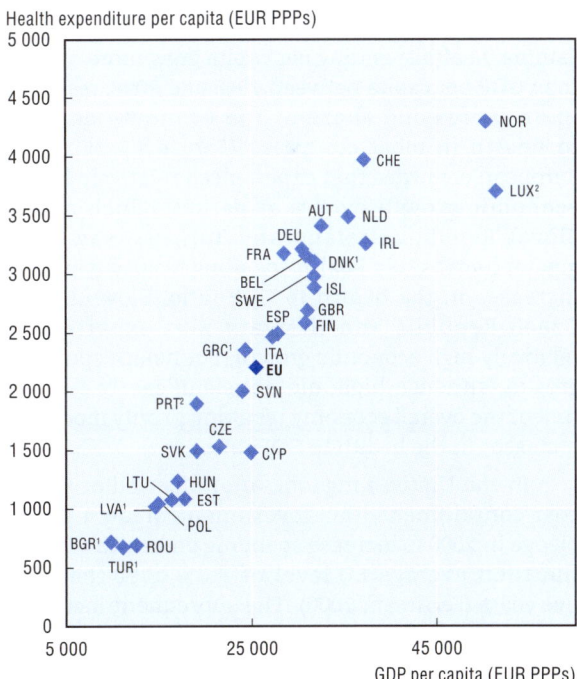

1. 2007. 2. 2006.
Source: OECD Health Data 2010; Eurostat Statistics Database; WHO National Health Accounts.

StatLink 🔗 *http://dx.doi.org/10.1787/888932337357*

In 2008, European Union countries devoted 8.3% of their GDP on average to health spending (Figure 4.2.1), up from 7.3% in 1998. The ratio of health spending to GDP among European countries in 2008 ranged from around 6% in Cyprus and Romania to more than 11% of GDP in France (Figure 4.2.1). This compares with 16% in the United States. Of the other European countries, Switzerland, Austria, Germany and Belgium all allocated more than 10% of their national economies to health spending.

In terms of public expenditure on health to GDP, European Union countries spent on average 6.2% of GDP, ranging from a high of 8.7% of GDP in France to lows of 2.4% and 4.1% in Cyprus and Turkey, respectively.

To get a more complete understanding of the key trends driving health spending, the health spending to GDP ratio should be considered together with per capita health spending. Countries having a relatively high health spending to GDP ratio might have relatively low health expenditure per capita, and the converse also holds. For example, Germany and Portugal both spent around 10% of their GDP on health; however, per capita spending (adjusted to EUR PPP) was more than 1.5 times higher in Germany (see Figure 4.1.1 from previous indicator).

Changes in the ratio of health spending to GDP are the result of the combined effect of growth in both GDP and health expenditure. Apart from Norway and Estonia, health spending per capita grew more quickly than GDP per capita between 1998 and 2008, resulting in an increasing share of the economy devoted to health in most countries (Figure 4.2.2). Some European countries that experienced relatively strong economic growth over that period – such as the Slovak Republic, Ireland and Turkey – saw even greater increases in health spending resulting in large increases in the health to GDP ratio. Slovenia, the Czech Republic and Hungary also experienced relatively high economic growth, but health spending growth, although high, did not significantly outpace that of the overall economy resulting in only moderate increases in the health to GDP ratio.

In the United Kingdom, after a period of strong cost containment, the government made a policy pledge in 2000 to increase spending on health to reach the then average EU level of 8.0% over the next five years (Ferriman, 2000). The subsequent increases in health spending meant that the United Kingdom

reached its target by 2004. At 8.7% in 2008, it is now slightly above the enlarged European Union member countries average (Figure 4.2.3).

As a result of the recession that started in many European countries in 2008 and became widespread in 2009, the ratio of health expenditure to GDP has increased sharply in some countries. In Ireland, the percentage of GDP devoted to health increased from 7.5% in 2007 to 8.7% in 2008, and in Spain from 8.4% to 9.0%. The share is likely to increase further when data for 2009 and 2010 become available as economic growth stalled or contracted while health spending growth continued. There is little evidence that GDP changes have an impact on the *level* of health spending in the short term. However, the experience of some European countries that have faced substantial recessions in the past 20 years is that health expenditures may be reduced in the following years as measures to reduce large public deficits are introduced (Scherer and Devaux, 2010).

In the long term, OECD projections of health and long-term care suggest that the drivers that have influenced health spending in the past such as rising incomes, technological changes and demographic factors will continue to exert upward pressures. The results indicate that public expenditure on health and long-term care as a share of GDP could almost double between 2005 and 2050 on average across OECD countries. Even if governments adopted more cost-containment policies, public health and long-term care spending would still increase by around 50% over the same period (OECD, 2006).

Definition and deviations

See Indicator 4.1 for the definition of total health expenditure.

Gross Domestic Product (GDP) = final consumption + gross capital formation + net exports. Final consumption of households includes goods and services used by households or the community to satisfy their individual needs. It includes final consumption expenditure of households, general government and non-profit institutions serving households.

4.2.1. Total health expenditure as a share of GDP, 2008

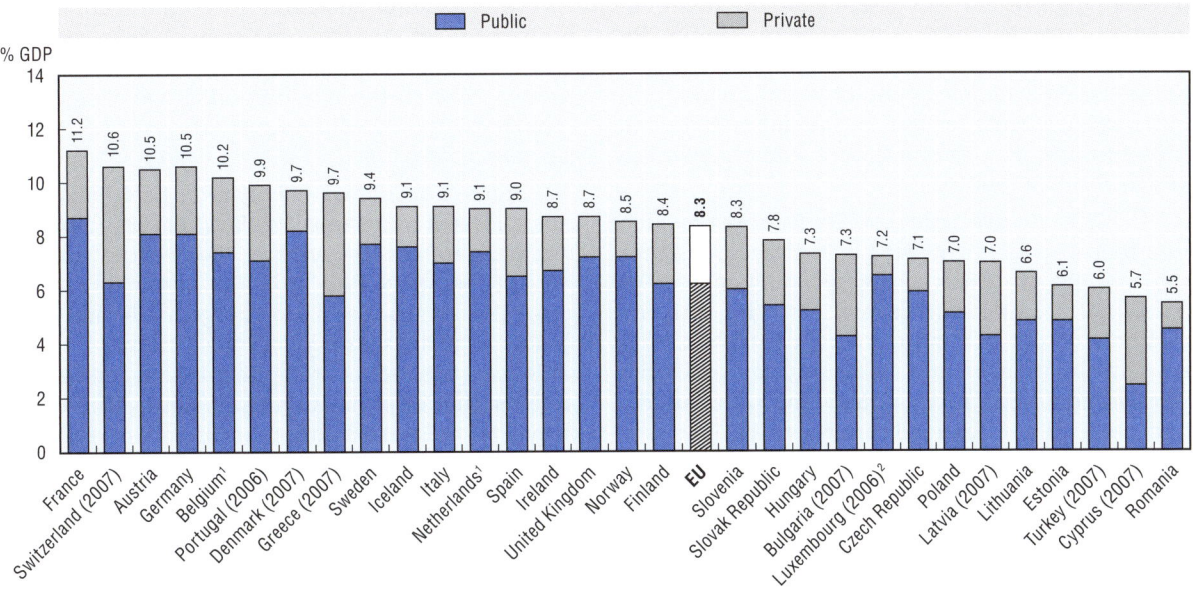

1. Public and private expenditures are current expenditures (excluding investments).
2. Health expenditure is for the insured population rather than resident population.

Source: OECD Health Data 2010; Eurostat Statistics Database; WHO National Health Accounts.

StatLink http://dx.doi.org/10.1787/888932337376

4.2.2. Annual average growth in real per capita expenditure on health and GDP, 1998-2008

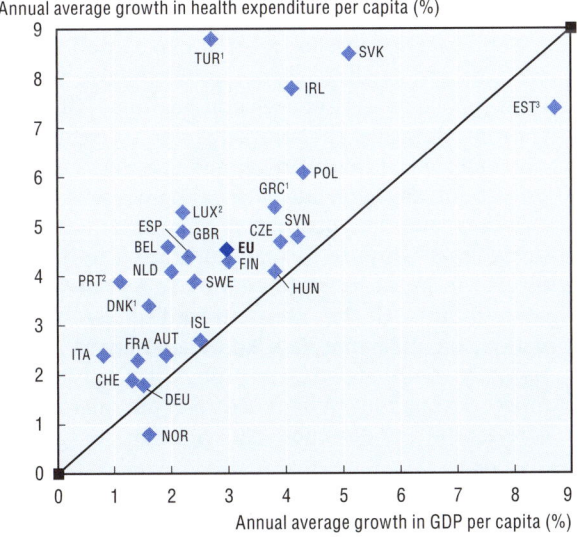

1. 1998-2007.   2. 1998-2006.   3. 1999-2007.

Source: OECD Health Data 2010; Eurostat Statistics Database; WHO National Health Accounts.

StatLink http://dx.doi.org/10.1787/888932337395

4.2.3. Total health expenditure as a share of GDP, 1998-2008

Selected EU countries

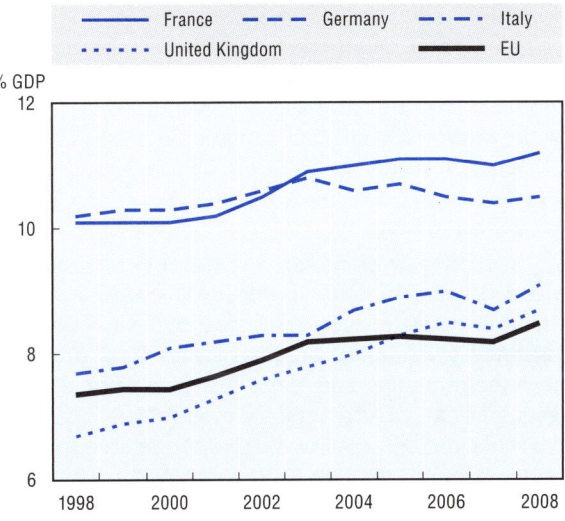

Source: OECD Health Data 2010; Eurostat Statistics Database; WHO National Health Accounts.

StatLink http://dx.doi.org/10.1787/888932337414

The allocation of health spending across the different types of health services and goods is influenced by a range of factors, including the availability of resources such as hospital beds, physicians and access to new technology, the financial and institutional arrangements for health care delivery, as well as by national clinical guidelines and the disease burden within a country.

In 2008, curative and rehabilitative care provided for either in-patients or out-patients accounted for just over 60% of current health spending on average across EU countries (Figure 4.3.1). The ratio of in-patient to out-patient spending depends on the institutional arrangements for health care provision. Austria and France, for example, report a relatively high proportion of expenditure for in-patient care (amounting to more than a third of total health spending) which is associated with a high level of hospital activity. Conversely, countries such as Portugal and Spain, with low levels of hospital activity, allocate only around a quarter of health care resources to in-patient care.

There are large differences between countries in their expenditure on long-term care. Norway and Denmark, with established formal arrangements for elderly care, allocate more than 20% of total health spending to long-term care. In Portugal, where care tends to be provided in more informal or family settings, the expenditure on long-term care accounts for a much smaller share of total spending.

The other major category of health expenditure is on medical goods, mostly accounted for by pharmaceuticals (see Indicator 4.4). On average, one-quarter of the share of health spending is on medical goods but it can be as low as 12-13% in Switzerland, Norway and Denmark, and as high as 38% in the Slovak Republic and Bulgaria.

Curative-rehabilitative care covers not only medical services requiring hospitalisation, but also those services provided as an out-patient or in a patient's own home. Changes in medical practice, new technologies and more efficient allocation of resources can all affect the balance between different types of care delivery. Day surgery is one area that has been expanding in many European countries in recent years.

The use of day surgery for procedures such as cataract removal (see Indicator 3.10) or hernia repairs may result in higher volumes and decreased unit costs. In many countries, day care has accounted for an increasing share of the total spending on curative care in recent years (Figure 4.3.2). There are, however, wide variations in spending, partly reflecting data

limitations, but also national policies and regulations. In France, spending on day care now accounts for around 11% of curative care spending. By contrast, Germany, where day surgery in public hospitals was prohibited until the late 1990s (Castoro et al., 2007), reported only 2% of curative care expenditure as services of day care.

Figure 4.3.3 shows the share of health expenditure allocated to organised public health and prevention programmes. On average, EU countries allocated 2.9% of their spending on health to a wide range of activities such as vaccination programmes and public health campaigns on alcohol abuse and smoking. The wide variation reflects to a great extent the national organisation of prevention campaigns. Where such initiatives are carried out at the primary care level, as in Spain, the prevention function is not captured separately and may be included under the spending on curative care. Other countries adopting a more centralised approach to public health and prevention campaigns are more able to identify spending on such programmes.

Definition and deviations

The functional approach of the *System of Health Accounts* (OECD, 2000) defines the boundaries of the health system. Current health expenditure comprises personal health care (curative care, rehabilitative care, long-term care, ancillary services and medical goods) and collective services (public health services and health administration). Curative, rehabilitative and long-term care can also be classified by mode of production (in-patient, day care, out-patient and home care). Day care comprises health care services delivered to patients who are formally admitted to hospitals, ambulatory premises or self standing centres but with the intention to discharge the patient on the same day. An out-patient is not formally admitted to a facility (physician's private office, hospital out-patient centre or ambulatory-care centre) and does not stay overnight.

Factors limiting the comparability across countries include estimations of long-term care expenditure. Also, expenditure in hospitals may be used as a proxy for in-patient care services, although hospital expenditure may include spending on out-patient, ancillary, and in some cases drug dispensing services (Orosz and Morgan, 2004).

4.3.1. Current health expenditure by function of health care, 2008

Countries are ranked by in-patient curative care as a share of current expenditure on health

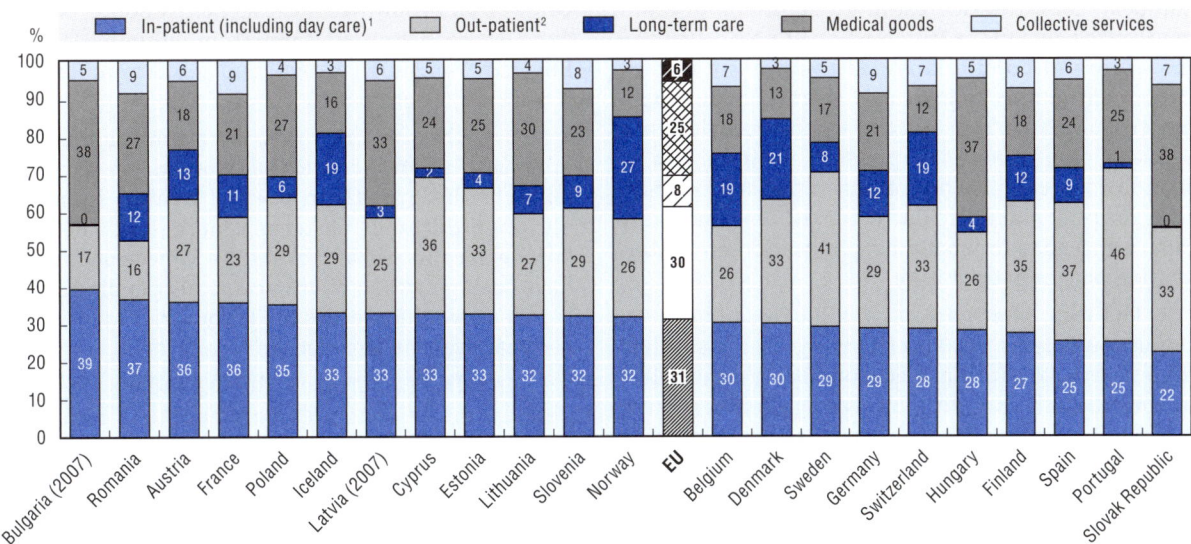

1. Refers to curative and rehabilitative in-patient and day care services provided in hospitals, day surgery clinics, etc.
2. Refers to curative and rehabilitative care in doctors' offices, clinics, out-patient departments of hospitals, home-care and ancillary services.

Source: OECD Health Data 2010; Eurostat Statistics Database.

StatLink http://dx.doi.org/10.1787/888932337433

4.3.2. Day care as a share of total curative care expenditure, 2004 and 2008

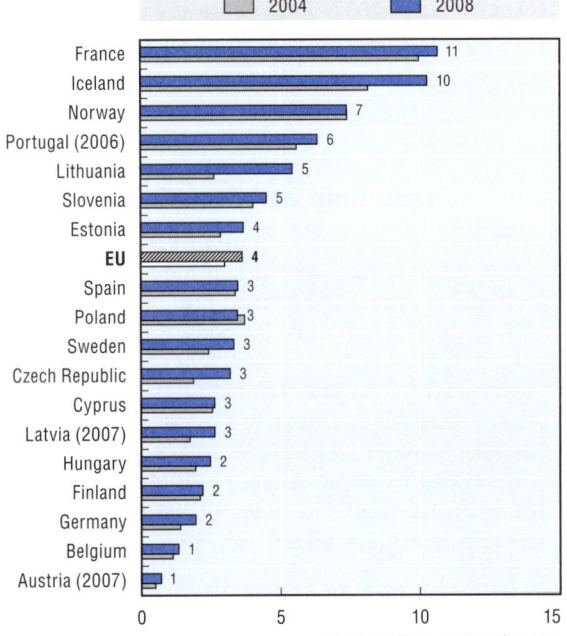

Note: Day care services provided in hospitals, day surgery clinics and other settings.

Source: OECD Health Data 2010; Eurostat Statistics Database.

StatLink http://dx.doi.org/10.1787/888932337452

4.3.3. Expenditure on organised public health and prevention programmes, 2008

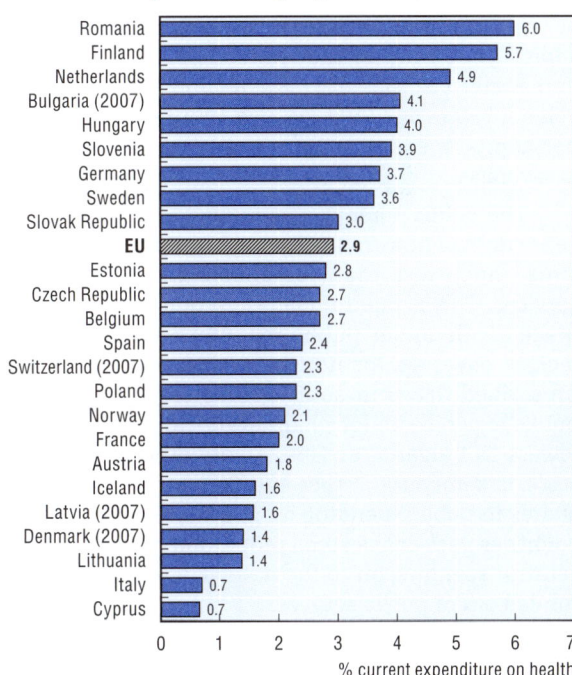

Source: OECD Health Data 2010; Eurostat Statistics Database.

StatLink http://dx.doi.org/10.1787/888932337471

Spending on pharmaceuticals account for a significant proportion of total health spending in European countries. Increased consumption of pharmaceuticals due to the introduction of new drugs and the ageing of populations has been an important factor contributing to increased overall heath expenditure (OECD, 2008a). However, the relationship between pharmaceutical spending and total health spending is a complex one, in that increased expenditure on pharmaceuticals to tackle diseases may reduce the need for costly hospitalisation and intervention now or in the future.

The total pharmaceutical bill across European Union countries in 2008 is estimated to have reached more than EUR 180 billion, accounting for around 18% of total health spending on average (unweighted) across EU countries. Over the past ten years, average spending per capita on pharmaceuticals has risen by almost 50% in real terms. However, considerable variation in pharmaceutical spending can be observed, reflecting differences in volume, structure of consumption and pharmaceutical pricing policies (Figure 4.4.1). Greece and Ireland spent the most per capita on pharmaceutical products, with spending of EUR 584 and EUR 563 respectively, compared with an EU average of EUR 376. Other countries that spent in excess of EUR 500 per capita on pharmaceutical products in 2008 were France, Belgium and Spain. At the other end of the scale, Romania spent just EUR 172 per capita – one-third of the French total. Other central and eastern European countries including Estonia, Poland, Latvia and Bulgaria also feature as the lowest per capita spenders at less than two-thirds of the EU average.

The public purse covers around 60% of pharmaceutical expenditure on average in European countries, much less than for physician and hospital services. This is due to higher co-payments for pharmaceuticals under public insurance schemes, or a lack of coverage for non-prescribed drugs and for prescribed drugs in some countries. The share of public expenditure for pharmaceutical drugs was the lowest in Bulgaria, at 20%. At the other end of the scale, Luxembourg, Greece and Germany all have high shares in public spending on pharmaceuticals. These countries pass only a small proportion of the pharmaceutical spending on to the patient, with around 80% funded out of public sources.

Pharmaceutical spending accounted for 1.7% of GDP on average across EU countries, ranging from below 1% in countries such as Luxembourg, Norway and Denmark, to more than 2% in Lithuania, Greece, Bulgaria, Hungary, Portugal and the Slovak Republic (Figure 4.4.1, right panel).

Over the past ten years, the average annual real growth in pharmaceutical spending has exceeded slightly the growth in overall health spending, although different patterns emerge both between European countries and over time. Greece and Ireland have seen growth in pharmaceutical spending significantly above the average of EU countries, at over 11% per year over the past decade (Figure 4.4.2).

Growth in pharmaceutical spending reached a peak in many countries between 1999 and 2001. Since then, policymakers have attempted to control pharmaceutical expenditures via a mix of price and volume controls directed at physicians and pharmacies, as well as policies targeting specific products (e.g. through product rebates) or increasing the share of cost borne by users. Recently, reductions in drug prices for reimbursed pharmaceuticals have been announced in Ireland, Greece and Sweden. Other initiatives encouraged greater use of cheaper generic alternatives, including through lower user co-payments, for example in Switzerland. The increased use of tendering for generics, in the Netherlands since 2005 and in Germany since 2007, has also allowed substantial savings in pharmaceutical spending (OECD, 2010b).

Definition and deviations

Pharmaceutical expenditure covers spending on prescription medicines and self-medication, often referred to as over-the-counter products, as well as other medical non-durable goods. It also includes pharmacists' remuneration when the latter is separate from the price of medicines. Pharmaceuticals consumed in hospitals are excluded (their inclusion would add another 15% to pharmaceutical spending approximately). Final expenditure on pharmaceuticals includes wholesale and retail margins and value-added tax.

4.4.1. Expenditure on pharmaceuticals per capita and as a share of GDP, 2008

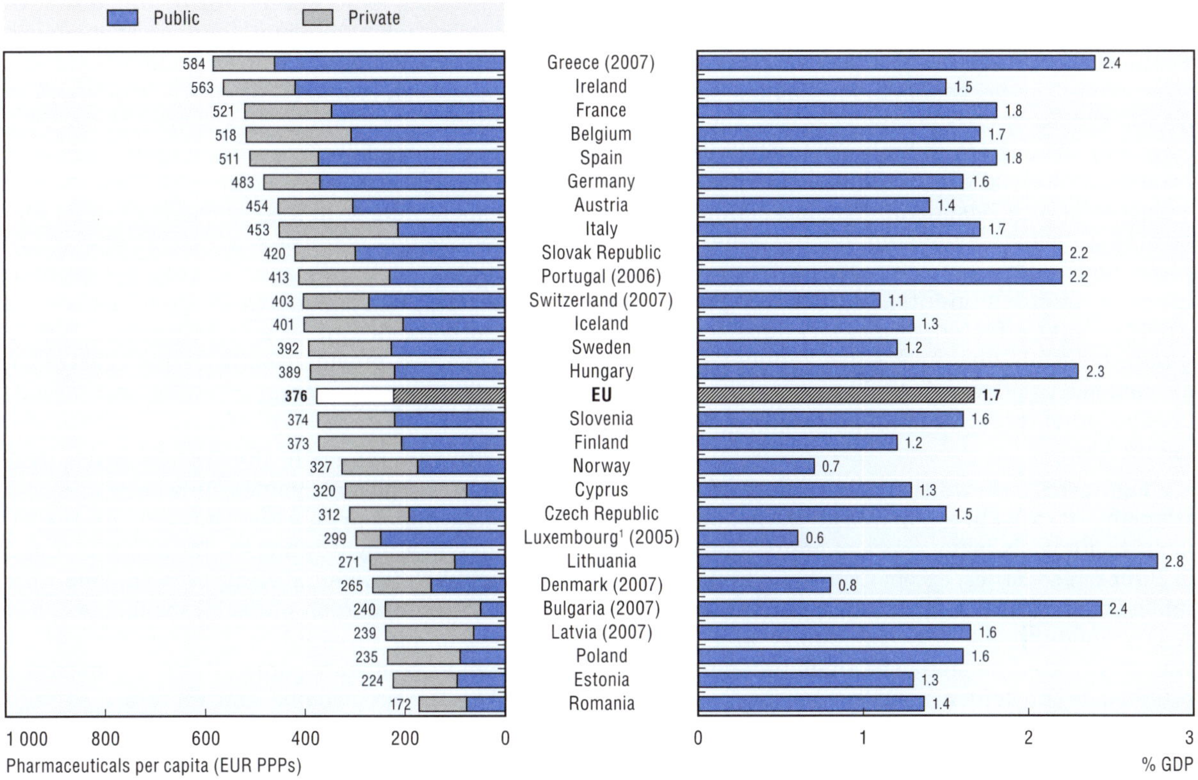

Public   Private

Country	Per capita (EUR PPPs)	% GDP
Greece (2007)	584	2.4
Ireland	563	1.5
France	521	1.8
Belgium	518	1.7
Spain	511	1.8
Germany	483	1.6
Austria	454	1.4
Italy	453	1.7
Slovak Republic	420	2.2
Portugal (2006)	413	2.2
Switzerland (2007)	403	1.1
Iceland	401	1.3
Sweden	392	1.2
Hungary	389	2.3
EU	**376**	**1.7**
Slovenia	374	1.6
Finland	373	1.2
Norway	327	0.7
Cyprus	320	1.3
Czech Republic	312	1.5
Luxembourg[1] (2005)	299	0.6
Lithuania	271	2.8
Denmark (2007)	265	0.8
Bulgaria (2007)	240	2.4
Latvia (2007)	239	1.6
Poland	235	1.6
Estonia	224	1.3
Romania	172	1.4

Pharmaceuticals per capita (EUR PPPs)   % GDP

1. Prescribed medicines only.

Source: OECD Health Data 2010; Eurostat Statistics Database; WHO National Health Accounts.

StatLink 🔗 *http://dx.doi.org/10.1787/888932337490*

4.4.2. Average annual real growth in pharmaceuticals expenditure compared to total health expenditure, 1998-2008

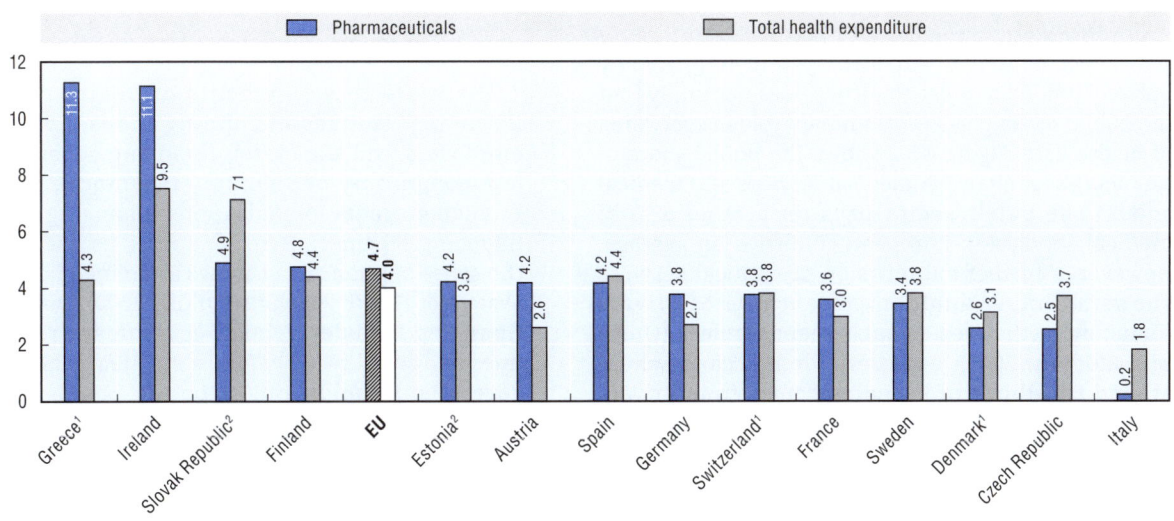

Pharmaceuticals   Total health expenditure

Country	Pharmaceuticals	Total health expenditure
Greece[1]	11.3	4.3
Ireland	11.1	9.5
Slovak Republic[2]	4.9	7.1
Finland	4.8	4.4
EU	4.7	4.0
Estonia[2]	4.2	3.5
Austria	4.2	2.6
Spain	4.2	4.4
Germany	3.8	2.7
Switzerland[1]	3.8	3.8
France	3.6	3.0
Sweden	3.4	3.8
Denmark[1]	2.6	3.1
Czech Republic	2.5	3.7
Italy	0.2	1.8

1. 1998-2007.
2. 1999-2008.

Source: OECD Health Data 2010; Eurostat Statistics Database.

StatLink 🔗 *http://dx.doi.org/10.1787/888932337509*

All European countries use a mix of public and private financing of health care, but to differing degrees. Public financing is confined to government revenues in countries where central and/or local governments are primarily responsible for financing health services directly (e.g. Sweden and the United Kingdom). It consists of both general government revenues and social contributions in countries with social insurance based-funding (e.g. France and Germany). Private financing, on the other hand, covers households' out-of-pocket payments (either direct or as co-payments), third-party payment arrangements effected through various forms of private health insurance, health services such as occupational health care directly provided by employers, and other direct benefits provided by charities and the like.

Figure 4.5.1 shows the public share of health financing across European countries in 2008. The public sector is the main source of health financing in all European countries, except Cyprus. On average, the public share of health spending was 73.6% in 2008. In Luxembourg, the Czech Republic, the Nordic countries (except Finland), the United Kingdom, the Netherlands and Romania, public financing accounted for more than 80% of all health expenditure. There has been a convergence of the public share of health spending among European countries over recent decades. Many of those countries with a relatively high public share in the early 1990s, such as Poland and Hungary, have decreased their share, while other countries which historically had a relatively low level (e.g. Portugal, Turkey) have increased their public share, reflecting health system reforms and the expansion of public coverage.

The fact that the health system is primarily publicly funded in most countries does not imply that the public sector plays the dominant role in every area of health care. Figure 4.5.2 shows the public share of financing separately for medical services and medical goods. The public sector pays for around 82% of medical services in European countries on average. However, a further sub-division of medical services shows an increasingly important role of private financing in the area of out-patient services (Orosz and Morgan, 2004), especially dental care, where around two-thirds of spending comes from private sources. In the financing of medical goods (pharmaceuticals and other goods), private payments also play an important role, most evident in Bulgaria, Latvia and Cyprus but also in other central and eastern European countries.

The size and composition of private financing for all health services and goods differs considerably across countries. On average, more than two-thirds of private funding is accounted for by out-of-pocket payments, including any cost-sharing arrangements (Colombo and Morgan, 2006). In some central and eastern European countries, the practice of unofficial supplementary payments means that the level of out-of-pocket spending is probably underestimated. Private health insurance is around 3-4% of total health expenditure on average across European Union countries (Figure 4.5.3). For some countries, it plays a significant financing role. It provides primary coverage for certain population groups in Germany. In France, private health insurance finances 13% of overall spending, providing both complementary and supplementary coverage in a public system with universal reach.

Health care reform in the Netherlands in 2006 resulted in the government heavily regulating the market for compulsory health insurance: insurers are obliged to accept anybody and the insurance premium is unrelated to individual risks. At the same time, the day-to-day operation of health insurance is now organised under private law (Schäfer et al., 2010). Because of its obligatory nature, this is considered as a social insurance scheme and therefore counted under public health spending, even though it is managed by private insurance corporations. Voluntary private health insurance accounts for around 6% of health spending in the Netherlands, and is used mainly to pay for complementary services such as dental care, glasses and physiotherapy (for people without recognised chronic conditions).

Definition and deviations

There are three elements of health care financing: sources of funding (households, employers and the state), financing schemes (e.g. compulsory or voluntary insurance), and financing agents (organisations managing the financing schemes). Here "financing" is used in the sense of financing schemes as defined in the System of Health Accounts (OECD, 2000). Public financing includes general government revenues and social security funds. Private financing covers households' out-of-pocket payments, private health insurance and other private funds (NGOs and private corporations). Out-of-pocket payments are expenditures borne directly by the patient. They include cost-sharing and, in certain countries, estimations of informal payments to health care providers.

4.5.1. Public share of total expenditure on health, 2008

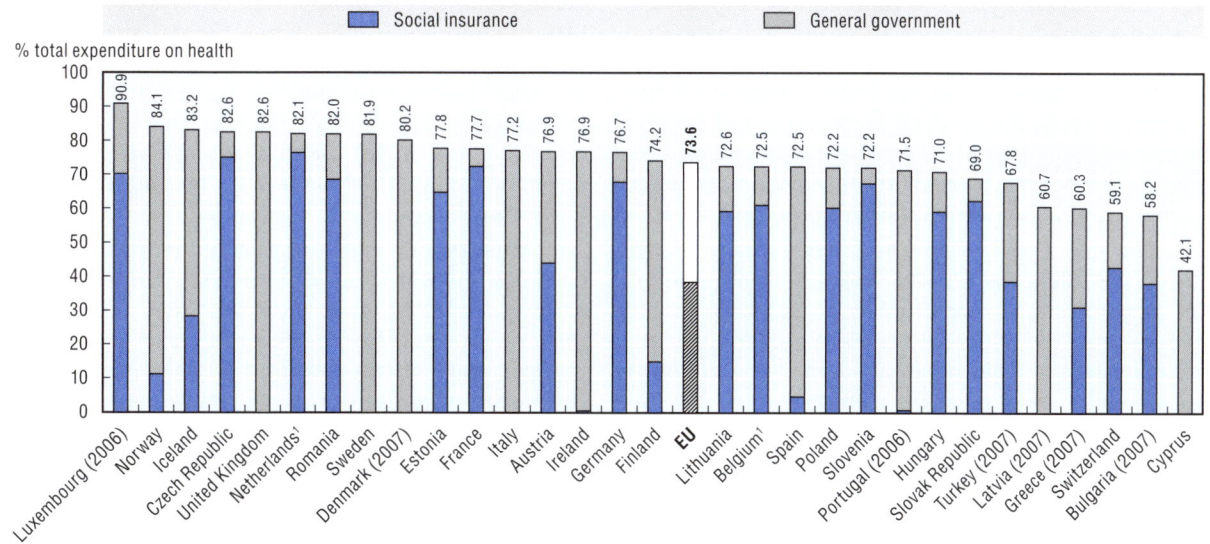

1. Share of current health expenditure.

Source: OECD Health Data 2010; Eurostat Statistics Database.

StatLink http://dx.doi.org/10.1787/888932337528

4.5.2. Public share of expenditure on medical services and goods, 2008

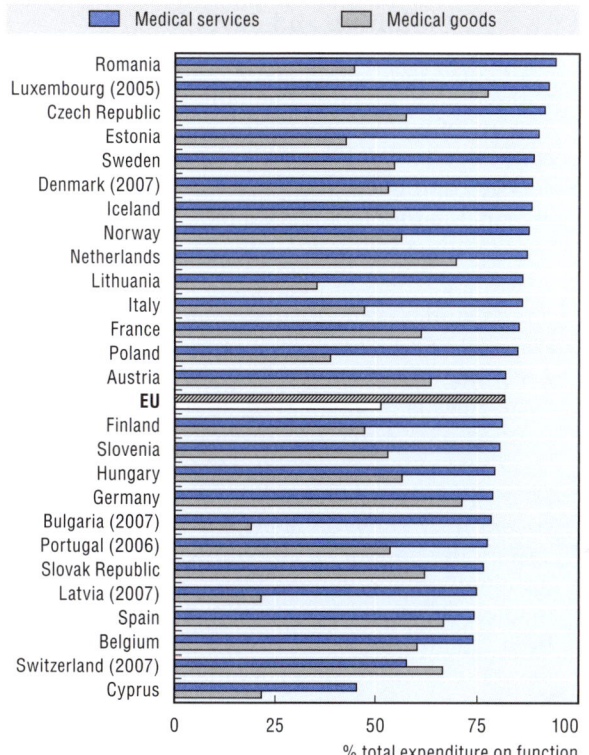

Source: OECD Health Data 2010; Eurostat Statistics Database.

StatLink http://dx.doi.org/10.1787/888932337547

4.5.3. Out-of-pocket and private health insurance expenditure, 2008

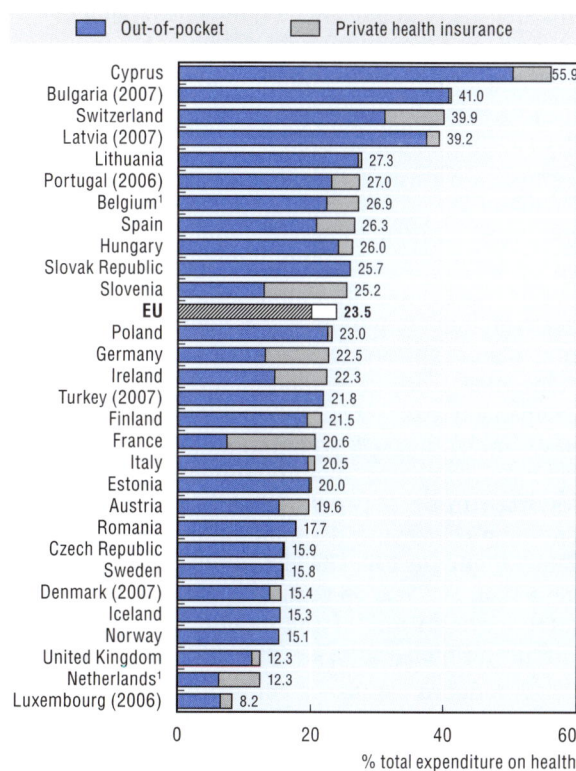

1. Current expenditure.

Source: OECD Health Data 2010; Eurostat Statistics Database.

StatLink http://dx.doi.org/10.1787/888932337566

The trend towards globalisation, reinforced by the relaxation of regulatory obstacles in Europe, has fuelled a steady growth in international trade in health services in recent years, albeit from relatively low levels. However, despite much attention from health analysts, the medical professions and health policy makers, discussions on the opportunities and challenges related to such trade have so far been conducted with relatively little data to inform them.

The major part of international trade in health services involves the physical movement of patients across borders to receive treatment – otherwise called patient mobility. While for the most part individuals prefer to receive health care in their home country, under certain circumstances it may be more beneficial to receive health care abroad; for example, where the nearest health facility may be across a border, when visiting a country as a tourist or on business, or if the required care can be provided faster, cheaper or of a higher quality. To get a full measure of imports and exports, there is also a need to consider goods and services delivered remotely such as pharmaceuticals ordered from another country or diagnostic services provided from a doctor in one country to a patient in another. The magnitude of such trade remains small, but advances in technology mean that this area also has the potential to grow rapidly.

Data on imports of health services and goods are available for the majority of European countries. They show that total reported imports amounted to more than EUR 3 billion in 2008 (Figure 4.6.1). The vast majority of this trade is between European countries. Germany is by far the greatest importer of health goods and services, partly reflecting a large growth in pharmaceuticals acquired from foreign-based on-line pharmacies in recent years. Other countries with relatively high imports are the Netherlands, France, Luxembourg and Belgium where much patient movement takes place in the border regions. However, in comparison to the size of the health sector as a whole, trade in health goods and services remains marginal for most countries. Even in the case of Germany, reported imports represent only around 0.5% of Germany's current health expenditure. Growth in the value of imports over the last five years has averaged more than 15% year on year, with much higher growth rates among some of the newer members of the European Union (Figure 4.6.2).

A reduced number of countries currently report exports of health services via international trade statistics totalling around EUR 2.5 billion (Figure 4.6.3). For both imports and exports, the figures are likely to be significant underestimates. The Czech Republic, France and Poland all reported exports in excess of EUR 400 million in 2008. Some central and eastern European countries have become popular destinations for patients from other European countries, particularly for services such as dental surgery. Annual growth has been over 30% in both the Czech Republic and Poland over the past five years (Figure 4.6.4).

Patient mobility in Europe could receive a further boost as the European Commission has sought to clarify patients' rights for treatment coverage in other member states. Many of the proposed changes in European regulations seek to strike a balance between the rights of patients to seek health care and the responsibilities of states to organise the delivery of health services. A Directive has been proposed, seeking to meet three objectives: to guarantee that all patients have care that is safe and of good quality; to support patients in the exercise of their rights to cross border health care; and to promote co-operation between health systems (Council of the European Union, 2010).

Definition and deviations

The *System of Health Accounts* includes imports within current health expenditure, defined as imports of medical goods and services for final consumption. Of these the purchase of medical services and goods, by resident patients while abroad, is currently the most important in value terms.

In the balance of payments, trade refers to goods and services transactions between residents and non-residents of an economy. According to the *Manual on Statistics of International Trade in Services*, "Health-related travel" is defined as "goods and services acquired by travellers going abroad for medical reasons". This category has some limitations in that it covers only those persons travelling for the specific purpose of receiving medical care, and does not include those who happen to require medical services when abroad. The additional item "Health services" covers those services delivered across borders but can include medical services delivered between providers as well as to patients.

4.6.1. Imports of health services and goods, 2003 and 2008

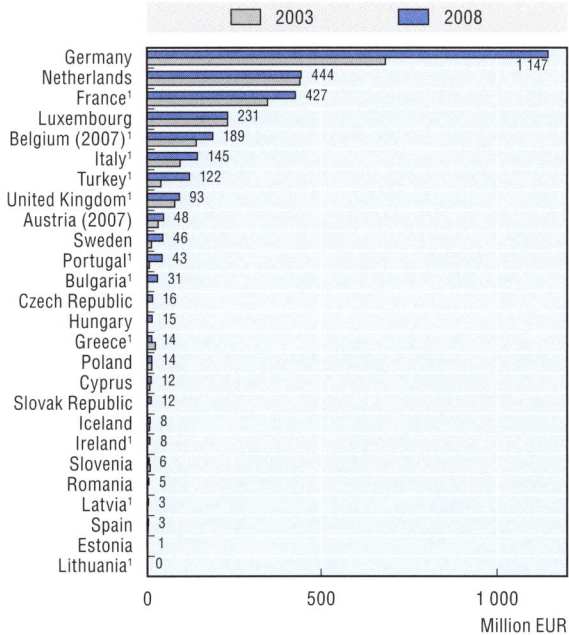

Note: Imports of health services and goods occur when residents receive medical services from foreign providers or when they purchase medical goods abroad.
1. Balance of payments concept of imports.
Source: OECD-Eurostat Trade in Services, OECD System of Health Accounts.

StatLink 〰⬛ http://dx.doi.org/10.1787/888932337585

4.6.3. Exports of health services and goods, 2003 and 2008

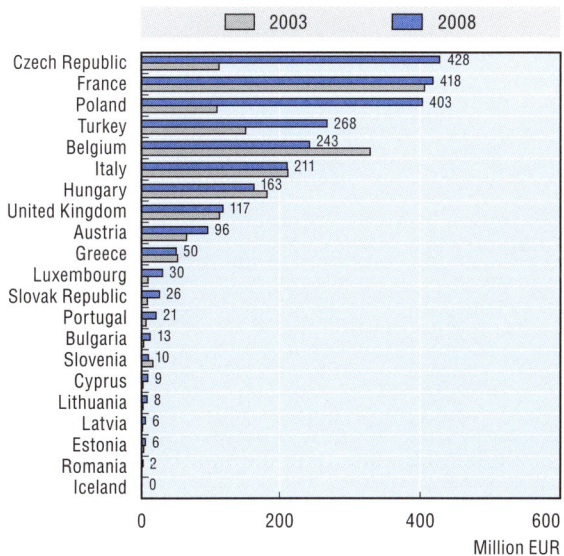

Note: Exports of health services and goods occur when domestic providers supply medical services to non-residents or when they sell medical goods to non-residents.
Source: OECD-Eurostat Trade in Services, OECD System of Health Accounts.

StatLink 〰⬛ http://dx.doi.org/10.1787/888932337623

4.6.2. Annual average growth rate in imports of health services and goods, 2003-08

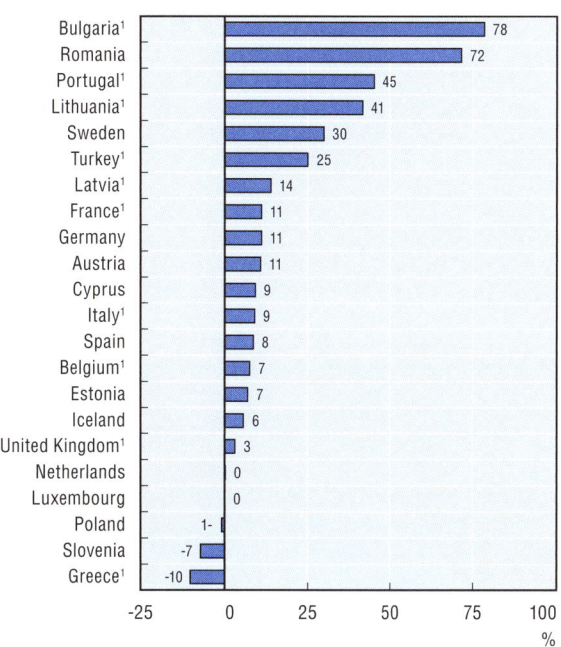

Note: Imports of health services and goods occur when residents receive medical services from foreign providers or when they purchase medical goods abroad.
1. Balance of payments concept of imports.
Source: OECD-Eurostat Trade in Services, OECD System of Health Accounts.

StatLink 〰⬛ http://dx.doi.org/10.1787/888932337604

4.6.4. Annual average growth rate in exports of health services and goods, 2003-08

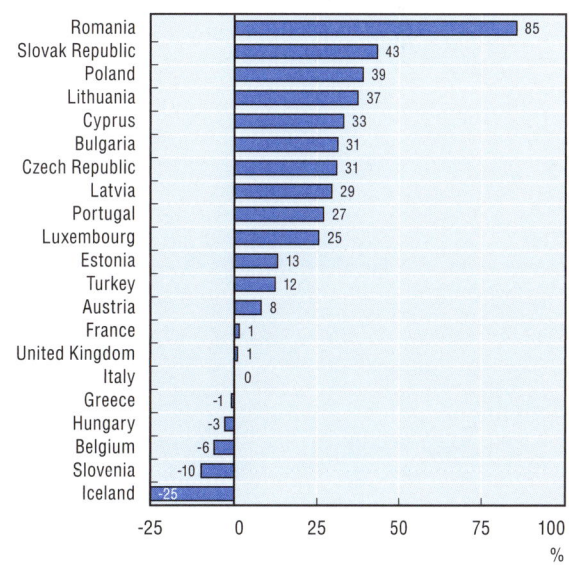

Note: Exports of health services and goods occur when domestic providers supply medical services to non-residents or when they sell medical goods to non-residents.
Source: OECD-Eurostat Trade in Services, OECD System of Health Accounts.

StatLink 〰⬛ http://dx.doi.org/10.1787/888932337642

Bibliography

Almasi, K. *et al.* (2009), "Risk Factors for Suicide in Hungary: A Case-control Study", *British Medical Journal Psychiatry*, Vol. 9, No. 45.

Alzheimer Europe (2009), "Cost of Illness and Burden of Dementia in Europe – Prognosis to 2030", *www.alzheimer-europe.org*.

Baert, K. and B. de Norre (2009), "Perception of Health and Access to Health Care in the EU-25 in 2007", *Eurostat Statistics in Focus 24/2009*, European Commission, Luxembourg.

Beck, L.F., A.M. Dellinger and M.E. O'Neil (2007), "Motor Vehicle Crash Injury Rates by Mode of Travel, United States: Using Exposure-based Methods to Quantify Differences", *American Journal of Epidemiology*, Vol. 166, pp. 212-218.

Bennett, J. (2003), "Investment in Population Health in Five OECD Countries", *OECD Health Working Papers*, No. 2, OECD Publishing, Paris.

Busse, R. and A. Riesberg (2004), *Health Care Systems in Transition: Germany*, WHO Regional Office for Europe on behalf of the European Observatory on Health Systems and Policies, Copenhagen.

Castoro, C. *et al.* (2007), *Policy Brief – Day Surgery: Making it Happen*, World Health Organisation on Behalf of the European Observatory on Health Systems and Policies, Copenhagen.

Cayotte, E. and H. Buchow (2009), "Who Dies of What in Europe Before the Age of 65", *Eurostat Statistics in Focus 67/2009*, European Commission, Luxembourg.

Chaloff, J. (2008), "Mismatches in the Formal Sector, Expansion of the Informal Sector: Immigration of Health Professionals to Italy", *OECD Health Working Papers*, No. 34, OECD Publishing, Paris.

Cole, T.J. *et al.* (2000), "Establishing a Standard Definition for Child Overweight and Obesity Worldwide: International Survey", *British Medical Journal*, Vol. 320, pp. 1-6.

Colombo, F. and D. Morgan (2006), "Evolution of Health Expenditure in OECD Countries", *Revue française des affaires sociales*, April-September.

Council of the European Union (2010), "Council Agrees on New Rules for Patients' Rights in Cross-border Healthcare", Press Release, PRESSE 10760/10, Luxembourg, 8 June 2010.

Currie, C. *et al.* (eds.) (2000), *Health and Health Behaviour among Young People (1997/98)*, WHO Regional Office for Europe, Copenhagen.

Currie, C. *et al.* (eds.) (2004), *Young People's Health in Context: International Report from the HBSC 2001/2002 Survey*, WHO Regional Office for Europe, Copenhagen.

Currie, C. *et al.* (eds.) (2008), *Inequalities in Young People's Health: Health Behaviour in School-aged Children (HBSC) International Report from the 2005/2006 Survey*, WHO Regional Office for Europe, Copenhagen.

Delamaire, M.L. and G. Lafortune (2010), "Nurses in Advanced Roles: A Description and Evaluation of Experiences in 12 Developed Countries", *OECD Working Papers*, No. 54, OECD Publishing, Paris.

Department of Health and Children (2001), "National Health Strategy: Quality and Fairness – A Health System for You", Stationery Office, Dublin.

Dormont, B. and H. Huber (2006), "Causes of Health Expenditure Growth: The Predominance of Changes in Medical Practices Over Population Ageing", *Annales d'Économie et de Statistique*, pp. 83-84, 187-217.

DREES (2009), "La démographie médicale à l'horizon 2030 : de nouvelles projections nationales et régionales", *Études et résultats*, No. 679, February.

ECDC (European Centre for Disease Prevention and Control)/WHO Regional Office for Europe (2009), *HIV/AIDS Surveillance in Europe 2008*, ECDC, Stockholm.

ECDC (2009), *Annual Epidemiological Report on Communicable Diseases in Europe 2009*, Revised Edition. ECDC, Stockholm.

ECHIM (2010), *European Community Health Indicators Monitoring*, *www.echim.org*.

ETSC (European Transport Safety Council) (2003), *Transport Safety Performance in the EU: A Statistical Overview*, ETSC, Brussels.

EURO-PERISTAT (2008), *European Perinatal Health Report*, EURO-PERISTAT Project with SCPE, EUROCAT, EURONEOSTAT, Paris.

European Commission (2006), *European Guidelines for Quality Assurance in Breast Cancer Screening and Diagnosis*, 4th edition, Luxembourg.

European Commission (2007), *White Paper on a Strategy for Europe on Nutrition, Overweight and Obesity-Related Health Issues*, COM(2007)279final, Commission of the European Communities, Brussels.

European Commission (2008a), *Hospital Data Project Phase 2*, Final Report, Luxembourg, November.

European Commission (2008b), *Major and Chronic Diseases – Report 2007*, EC Directorate-General for Health and Consumers, Luxembourg.

European Commission (2008c), *European Guidelines for Quality Assurance in Cervical Cancer Screening*, 2nd edition, Luxembourg.

European Commission (2010a), *ECHI*, Factsheet, *http://ec.europa.eu/health/indicators/echi/list/index_en.htm*.

European Commission (2010b), "EU Actions on Information on Alzheimer and Other Dementias", *http://ec.europa.eu/health/major_chronic_diseases/diseases/brain_neurological/index_en.htm*.

European Commission (2010c), *Pandemic (H1N1) 2009, Factsheet*, EC Directorate-General for Health and Consumers, Luxembourg, April 2010.

European Union (2003), "Council Recommendation of 2 December 2003 on Cancer Screening (2003/879/EC)", *Official Journal of the European Union*, No. L327, Vol. 46, 16 December 2003, pp. 34-38.

EUVAC.NET (2009), *Measles Surveillance Annual Report 2008*, EUVAC.NET, Copenhagen.

EUVAC.NET (2010), *Pertussis Surveillance Annual Report 2008*, EUVAC.NET, Copenhagen.

Ferlay, J. *et al.* (2007), "Estimates of the Cancer Incidence and Mortality in Europe in 2006", *Annals of Oncology*, Vol. 18, pp. 581-592.

Ferlay, J. *et al.* (2010), *GLOBOCAN 2008, Cancer Incidence and Mortality Worldwide*, IARC CancerBase, No. 10 (Internet), International Agency for Research on Cancer, Lyon, available from: *http://globocan.iarc.fr*.

Ferriman, A. (2000), "Blair Will Have Difficulty in Matching European Spending", *British Medical Journal*, Vol. 320, No. 7230.

Foresight (2007), "Tackling Obesities: Future Choices", Government Office for Science, *www.foresight.gov.uk/Obesity/17.pdf*.

Fujisawa, R. and G. Lafortune (2008), "The Remuneration of General Practitioners and Specialists in 14 OECD Countries: What are the Factors Explaining Variations Across Countries", *OECD Health Working Papers*, No. 41, OECD Publishing, December.

Gatta, G. *et al.* (2000), "Toward a Comparison of Survival in American and European Cancer Patients", *Cancer*, Vol. 89, No. 4, pp. 893-900.

Hallal, P.C. *et al.* (2006), "Adolescent Physical Activity and Health: A Systematic Review", *Sports Medicine*, Vol. 36, No. 12, pp. 1019-1030.

Hawton, K. and K. van Heeringen (2009), "Suicide", *The Lancet*, Vol. 373, pp. 1373-1381.

Huang, C.M. (2008), "Human Papillomavirus and Vaccination", *Mayo Clinic Proceedings*, Vol. 83, No. 6, pp. 701-707.

IARC (2008), *World Cancer Report 2008*, IARC Press, Lyon.

IDF (International Diabetes Federation) (2006), *Diabetes Atlas*, 3rd edition, IDF, Brussels.

IDF (2009), *Diabetes Atlas*, 4th edition, IDF, Brussels.

Institute of Alcohol Studies (2007), "Binge Drinking-Nature, Prevalence and Causes", *IAS Fact Sheet*, *www.ias.org.uk/resources/factsheets/binge_drinking.pdf*.

Institute of Cancer Research (2009), "Prostate Cancer", *Fact Sheet*, *www.icr.ac.uk/everyman/about/prostate.html*.

Jagger, C. et al. (2008), "Inequalities in Healthy Life Years in the 25 Countries of the European Union in 2005: A Cross-national Meta-regression Analysis", *The Lancet*, Vol. 372, No. 9656, pp. 2124-2131.

Jagger, C. et al. (2010), "The Global Activity Limitation Indicator (GALI) Measured Function and Disability Similarly across European Countries", *Journal of Clinical Epidemiology*, Vol. 63, pp. 892-899.

Jha, P. et al. (2006), "Social Inequalities in Male Mortality, and in Male Mortality from Smoking: Indirect Estimation from National Death Rates in England and Wales, Poland, and North America", *The Lancet*, Vol. 368, No. 9533, pp. 367-370.

Joumard, I., C. Andre, C. Nicq and O. Chatal (2008), "Health Status Determinants: Lifestyle, Environment, Health Care Resources and Efficiency", *Economics Department Working Papers*, No. 627, OECD Publishing, Paris.

Kiely, J., K. Brett, S. Yu and D. Rowley (1995), "Low Birth Weight and Intrauterine Growth Retardation", in L. Wilcox and J. Marks (eds.), *From Data to Action: CDC's Public Health Surveillance for Women, Infants, and Children*, Center for Disease Control and Preventions, Atlanta, pp. 185-202.

King, H., R.E. Aubert and W.H. Herman (1998), "Global Burden of Diabetes, 1995-2025: Prevalence, Numerical Estimates, and Projections", *Diabetes Care*, Vol. 21, No. 9, pp. 1414-1431.

Koechlin, F., L. Lorenzoni and P. Schreyer (2010), "Comparing Price Levels of Hospital Services Across Countries: Results of a Pilot Study", *OECD Health Working Papers*, No. 53, OECD Publishing, Paris.

Kunze, U. et al. (2007), "Influenza Vaccination in Austria, 1982-2003", *Wien Med Wochenschr*, Vol. 157, No. 5-6, pp. 98-101.

Mackenbach, J.P. et al. (2008), "Socioeconomic Inequalities in Health in 22 European Countries", *New England Journal of Medicine*, Vol. 358, pp. 2468-2481.

Martinez-Palou, A. and E. Rohner-Thielen (2008), "Fruit and Vegetables: Fresh and Healthy on European Tables", *Eurostat Statistics in Focus 60/2008*, European Commission, Luxembourg.

Mathers, C. et al. (2005), "Counting the Dead and What They Died From: An Assessment of the Global Status of Cause of Death Data", *Bulletin of the World Health Organization*, Vol. 83, No. 3, pp. 171-177.

Mauri, D., N.P. Polyzos et al. (2008), "Multiple-Treatments Meta-Analysis of Chemotherapy and Targeted Therapies in Advanced Breast Cancer", *Journal of the National Cancer Institute*, Vol. 100, No. 24, pp. 1745-1747.

Miilunpalo, S. et al. (1997), "Self-rated Health Status as a Health Measure: the Predictive Value of Self-reported Health Status on the Use of Physician Services and on Mortality in the Working-age Population", *Journal of Clinical Epidemiology*, Vol. 50, pp. 90-93.

Moïse, P. (2003), "The Heart of the Health Care System: Summary of the Ischaemic Heart Disease Part of the OECD Ageing-related Diseases Study", *A Disease-based Comparison of Health Systems: What is Best and at What Cost?*, OECD Publishing, Paris.

Moïse, P. et al. (2003), "OECD Study of Cross-national Differences in the Treatment, Costs and Outcomes for Ischaemic Heart Disease", *OECD Health Working Papers*, No. 3, OECD Publishing, Paris.

Moon, L. et al. (2003), "Stroke Care in OECD Countries: A Comparison of Treatment, Costs and Outcomes in 17 OECD Countries", *OECD Health Working Papers*, No. 5, OECD Publishing, Paris.

NICE (2009), *Evaluation Pathway Programme for Medical Technologies*, London and Manchester.

NOMESCO (2007), *Health Statistics in the Nordic Countries 2005*, NOMESCO, Copenhagen.

OECD (2000), *A System of Health Accounts*, OECD Publishing, Paris.

OECD (2003), *A Disease-based Comparison of Health Systems: What is Best and at What Cost?*, OECD Publishing, Paris.

OECD (2004), *Towards High-Performing Health Systems*, OECD Publishing, Paris.

OECD (2005), *OECD Reviews of Health Systems – Finland*, OECD Publishing, Paris.

OECD (2006), "Projecting OECD Health and Long-term Care Expenditures: What Are the Main Drivers?", *OECD Economics Department Working Paper*, No. 477, OECD Publishing, Paris.

OECD (2008a), *Pharmaceutical Pricing Policies in a Global Market*, OECD Publishing, Paris.

OECD (2008b), *The Looming Crisis in the Health Workforce: How Can OECD Countries Respond?*, OECD Publishing, Paris.

OECD (2009), *OECD Economic Surveys: Greece*, OECD Publishing, Paris.

OECD (2010a), *OECD Health Data 2010*, on line and on CD-ROM, OECD Publishing, Paris.

OECD (2010b), *Health System Priorities when Money Is Tight*, OECD Publishing, Paris.

OECD (2010c), *Obesity and the Economics of Prevention: Fit not Fat*, OECD Publishing, Paris.

OECD and WHO (2006), *OECD Reviews of Health Systems – Switzerland*, OECD Publishing, Paris.

OECD and WHO (2010), "International Migration of Health Workers", Joint OECD-WHO Policy Brief, OECD, Paris.

OECD/ITF (International Transport Forum) (2008), *Trends in the Transport Sector 1970-2006*, OECD/ITF, Paris.

Orosz, E. and D. Morgan (2004), "SHA-Based National Health Accounts in Thirteen OECD Countries: A Comparative Analysis", *OECD Health Working Papers*, No. 16, OECD Publishing, Paris.

Paris, V. *et al.* (2010), "Health Systems Institutional Characteristics: A Survey of 29 OECD Countries", *OECD Health Working Papers*, No. 50, OECD Publishing, Paris.

Peden, M. *et al.* (eds.) (2004), *World Report on Road Traffic Injury Prevention*, World Health Organization, Geneva.

Rasmussen, M. *et al.* (2006), "Determinants of Fruit and Vegetable Consumption among Children and Adolescents: A Review of the Literature. Part 1: Quantitative Studies", *International Journal of Behavioral Nutrition and Physical Activity*, Vol. 3, No. 22.

Rehm, J. *et al.* (2009), "Global Burden of Disease and Injury and Economic Cost Attributable to Alcohol Use and Alcohol-use Disorder", *The Lancet*, Vol. 373, pp. 2223-2233.

Retzlaff-Roberts, D., C. Chang and R. Rubin (2004), "Technical Efficiency in the Use of Health Care Resources: A Comparison of OECD Countries", *Health Policy*, Vol. 69, pp. 55-72.

RIVM (National Institute for Public Health and the Environment) (2008), *Dare to Compare! Benchmarking Dutch Health with the European Community Health Indicators (ECHI)*, Bilthoven.

Sandvik, C. *et al.* (2005), "Personal, Social and Environmental Factors Regarding Fruit and Vegetable Consumption Intake among Schoolchildren in Nine European Countries", *Annals of Nutrition and Metabolism*, Vol. 49, No. 4, pp. 255-266.

Sassi, F., M. Devaux, M. Cecchini and E. Rusticelli (2009), "The Obesity Epidemic: Analysis of Past and Projected Future Trends in Selected OECD Countries", *OECD Health Working Papers*, No. 45, OECD Publishing, Paris.

Schäfer, W. *et al.* (2010), *Health Systems in Transition: The Netherlands Health System Review*, WHO Regional Office for Europe on behalf of the European Observatory on Health Systems and Policies, Vol. 12, No. 1, Copenhagen.

Secretary of State for Health (2002), *Delivering the NHS Plan: Next Steps on Investment, Next Steps on Reform*, The Stationery Office, London.

Scherer, P. and M. Devaux (2010), "The Challenge of Financing Health Care in the Current Crisis", *OECD Health Working Paper*, No. 49, OECD Publishing, Paris.

Shafey, O. *et al.* (eds.) (2009), *The Tobacco Atlas*, 3rd edition, American Cancer Society, Atlanta.

Sullivan, D.F. (1971), "A Single Index of Mortality and Morbidity", *Health Services Mental Health Administration Health Reports*, Vol. 86, pp. 347-354.

Swedish Association of Local Authorities and Regions and National Board of Health and Welfare (2008), *Quality and Efficiency in Swedish Health Care – Regional Comparisons 2008*, Stockholm.

Taggart, D. (2009), "PCI or CABG in Coronary Artery Disease?", *The Lancet*, Vol. 373, pp. 1190-1197.

Thompson, D. and A.M. Wolf (2001), "The Medical-Care Burden of Obesity", *Obesity Reviews*, No. 2, International Association for the Study of Obesity, pp. 189-197.

UNAIDS – Joint United Nations Programme in HIV/AIDS (2008), *Report on the Global HIV/AIDS Epidemic 2008*, UNAIDS, Geneva.

UNICEF and WHO (2004), *Low Birthweight: Country, Regional and Global Estimates*, UNICEF, New York.

Verdecchia, A. *et al.* (2007), "Recent Cancer Survival in Europe: A 2000-02 Period Analysis of EUROCARE-4 Data", *The Lancet Oncology*, Vol. 8, pp. 784-796.

WHO (World Health Organization) (1996), *Health Behaviour in School-aged Children: A World Health Organisation Cross-national Study (1993/94)*, WHO Regional Office for Europe, Copenhagen.

WHO (2000), "Obesity: Preventing and Managing the Global Epidemic. Report of a WHO Consultation", *WHO Technical Report Series*, No. 894, WHO, Geneva.

WHO (2004), *WHO Global Status Report on Alcohol 2004*, WHO, Geneva.

WHO (2009a), *Hepatitis B WHO Fact Sheet*, No. 204, WHO, Geneva.

WHO (2009b), *Global Status Report on Road Safety: Time for Action*, WHO, Geneva.

WHO (2010a), *Chronic Rheumatic Conditions, Fact Sheet, www.who.int/chp/topics/rheumatic/en/*, WHO, Geneva.

WHO (2010b), *World Health Statistics 2010*, WHO, Geneva.

WHO (2010c), *Management of Substance Abuse, www.who.int/substance_abuse/activities/globalstrategy/en/index.html*.

WHO Europe (2010), *Centralized Information System for Infectious Diseases*, Online: *data.euro.who.int/cisid/*

Woods, L.M., B. Rachet and M.P. Coleman (2006), "Origins of Socio-economic Inequalities in Cancer Survival: A Review", *Annals of Oncology*, Vol. 17, No. 1, pp. 5-19.

World Bank (1999), *Curbing the Epidemic: Governments and the Economics of Tobacco Control*, World Bank, Washington.

ANNEX A

Additional Information on Demographic and Economic Context

Table A.1. **Total population, thousands, 1960 to 2008**

	1960	1970	1980	1990	2000	2008
Austria	7 048	7 467	7 549	7 678	8 012	8 333
Belgium	9 154	9 656	9 859	9 967	10 251	10 517
Bulgaria	7 829	8 464	8 846	8 767	8 191	7 640
Cyprus	572	612	510	573	690	789
Czech Republic	9 660	9 805	10 327	10 363	10 273	10 262
Denmark	4 580	4 929	5 123	5 141	5 337	5 489
Estonia	1 216	1 365	1 473	1 567	1 370	1 341
Finland	4 430	4 606	4 780	4 986	5 176	5 307
France	45 684	50 772	53 880	56 709	59 049	61 840
Germany[1]	55 585	60 651	61 566	63 254	82 212	82 110
Greece	8 327	8 793	9 643	10 161	10 917	11 218
Hungary	9 984	10 338	10 711	10 374	10 211	10 035
Iceland	176	204	228	255	281	319
Ireland	2 832	2 950	3 401	3 506	3 790	4 250
Italy	50 200	53 822	56 434	56 719	56 942	58 863
Latvia	2 104	2 352	2 509	2 668	2 382	2 271
Lithuania	2 756	3 119	3 404	3 694	3 512	3 366
Luxembourg	314	340	364	382	436	471
Malta	327	303	315	352	380	410
Netherlands	11 487	13 039	14 150	14 952	15 926	16 390
Norway	3 581	3 876	4 086	4 241	4 491	4 768
Poland	29 383	32 622	35 578	38 031	38 258	38 116
Portugal	8 858	8 680	9 766	9 983	10 226	10 620
Romania	18 319	20 140	22 133	23 211	22 455	21 529
Slovak Republic	3 994	4 528	4 984	5 298	5 401	5 393
Slovenia	1 580	1 670	1 832	1927	1985	2015
Spain	30 455	33 753	37 527	38 851	40 264	44 311
Sweden	7 485	8 043	8 310	8 559	8 872	9 217
Switzerland	5 328	6 181	6 319	6 712	7 184	7 648
Turkey	27 438	35 294	44 522	56 104	67 393	74 768
United Kingdom	52 373	55 632	56 330	57 237	58 886	60 520
EU27	**386 536**	**418 451**	**441 304**	**454 910**	**481 404**	**492 623**

Break in series.

1. Note that population figures for Germany prior to 1991 refer to West Germany.

Source: OECD Reference Series (accessed in May 2010) and *Eurostat Statistics Database* (accessed in July 2010).

StatLink ⫘ http://dx.doi.org/10.1787/888932337661

Table A.2. **Share of the population aged 65 and over, 1960 to 2008**

	1960	1970	1980	1990	2000	2008
Austria	12.2	14.1	15.4	14.9	15.4	17.1
Belgium	12.0	13.4	14.3	14.9	16.8	17.3
Bulgaria	7.4	9.4	11.8	13.0	16.2	17.3
Cyprus[1]	. .	. .	10.8	10.8	11.2	12.5
Czech Republic	9.6	12.1	13.5	12.5	13.8	14.7
Denmark	10.6	12.3	14.4	15.6	14.8	15.7
Estonia	10.5	11.7	12.5	11.6	15.1	17.0
Finland	7.3	9.2	12.0	13.4	14.9	16.6
France	11.6	12.9	13.9	14.0	16.1	16.5
Germany	10.8	13.2	15.5	15.3	16.4	20.2
Greece	8.1	11.1	13.1	13.8	16.6	18.6
Hungary	9.0	11.6	13.4	13.3	15.1	16.3
Iceland	8.1	8.8	9.9	10.6	11.6	11.5
Ireland	11.1	11.1	10.7	11.4	11.2	11.5
Italy	9.3	10.9	13.1	14.9	18.3	20.3
Latvia	. .	11.9	13.0	11.8	14.8	17.2
Lithuania	. .	10.0	11.3	10.8	13.7	15.8
Luxembourg	10.8	12.5	13.6	13.4	14.1	14.5
Malta	. .	. .	8.4	10.4	12.1	13.5
Netherlands	9.0	10.2	11.5	12.8	13.6	14.9
Norway	11.0	12.9	14.8	16.3	15.2	14.7
Poland	6.0	8.4	10.1	10.1	12.2	13.5
Portugal	7.9	9.4	11.3	13.4	16.2	16.9
Romania	. .	8.5	10.3	10.3	13.4	14.9
Slovak Republic	6.9	9.2	10.5	10.3	11.4	12.4
Slovenia	7.8	9.9	11.4	11.1	14.0	16.0
Spain	8.2	9.6	11.2	13.6	16.8	17.0
Sweden	11.8	13.7	16.3	17.8	17.3	17.6
Switzerland	10.2	11.4	13.8	14.6	15.3	16.5
Turkey	3.6	4.4	4.7	4.4	5.4	6.1
United Kingdom	11.7	13.0	15.0	15.7	15.8	15.7
EU27	. .	. .	**12.5**	**13.0**	**14.7**	**16.0**

1. Data for Cyprus in 1980 refers to 1982.
Source: OECD Reference Series (accessed in May 2010) and *Eurostat Statistics Database* (accessed in July 2010).

StatLink ᵐˢᵖ http://dx.doi.org/10.1787/888932337680

Table A.3. **Crude birth rate, per 1 000 population, 1960 to 2008**

	1960	1970	1980	1990	2000	2008
Austria	17.9	15.0	12.1	11.8	9.8	9.3
Belgium	16.9	14.7	12.6	12.4	11.2	11.7
Bulgaria	17.8	16.3	14.5	12.1	9.0	10.2
Cyprus[1]	26.2	19.2	20.3	18.3	12.2	11.6
Czech Republic	13.3	15.1	14.9	12.6	8.8	11.7
Denmark	16.6	14.4	11.1	12.3	12.6	11.8
Estonia	16.6	15.8	15.1	14.2	9.5	12.0
Finland	18.5	14.1	13.2	13.2	11.0	11.3
France	17.9	16.7	14.8	13.4	13.1	13.0
Germany	17.4	13.4	10.1	11.5	9.3	8.3
Greece	18.9	16.5	15.3	10.1	9.5	10.5
Hungary	14.6	14.7	13.9	12.1	9.6	9.9
Iceland	27.9	19.6	19.7	18.8	15.4	15.2
Ireland	21.5	21.7	21.8	15.1	14.3	17.0
Italy	18.4	17.0	11.7	10.2	9.5	9.6
Latvia	16.7	14.6	14.1	14.2	8.5	10.6
Lithuania	22.5	17.7	15.2	15.4	9.8	10.4
Luxembourg	15.9	12.9	11.5	12.8	13.1	11.9
Malta	26.2	17.6	17.7	15.2	11.5	10.0
Netherlands	20.8	18.3	12.8	13.2	13.0	11.3
Norway	17.3	16.8	12.5	14.4	13.1	12.6
Poland	22.8	16.8	19.6	14.4	9.9	10.9
Portugal	24.2	20.9	16.2	11.6	11.7	9.8
Romania	19.1	21.1	17.9	13.6	10.4	10.3
Slovak Republic	22.1	17.8	19.1	15.1	10.2	10.8
Slovenia	17.6	16.4	16.3	11.6	9.2	10.8
Spain	21.7	19.6	15.2	10.3	9.9	11.4
Sweden	13.6	13.7	11.7	14.5	10.1	11.8
Switzerland	17.7	16.1	11.7	12.5	10.9	10.0
Turkey[2]	..	35.2	31.7	25.2	20.2	17.8
United Kingdom	17.5	16.2	13.4	14.0	11.5	12.9
EU27	**19.0**	**16.6**	**14.9**	**13.2**	**10.7**	**11.1**

1. Data for Cyprus in 1960 refers to 1961.
2. Data for Turkey in 1970 refers to 1973.
Source: OECD Health Data 2010 and Eurostat Statistics Database.

StatLink 🔗 *http://dx.doi.org/10.1787/888932337699*

Table A.4. **Fertility rate, number of children per women aged 15-49, 1960 to 2008**

	1960	1970	1980	1990	2000	2008
Austria	2.7	2.3	1.7	1.5	1.4	1.4
Belgium	2.5	2.3	1.7	1.6	1.7	1.8
Bulgaria	2.3	2.2	2.1	1.8	1.3	1.5
Cyprus[1]	..	..	2.5	2.4	1.6	1.5
Czech Republic	2.1	1.9	2.1	1.9	1.1	1.5
Denmark	2.5	2.0	1.6	1.7	1.8	1.9
Estonia	..	..	2.0	2.1	1.4	1.7
Finland	2.7	1.8	1.6	1.8	1.7	1.9
France	2.7	2.5	2.0	1.8	1.9	2.0
Germany	2.4	2.0	1.6	1.5	1.4	1.4
Greece	2.3	2.4	2.2	1.4	1.3	1.5
Hungary	2.0	2.0	1.9	1.8	1.3	1.4
Iceland	4.3	2.8	2.5	2.3	2.1	2.1
Ireland	3.8	3.9	3.2	2.1	1.9	2.1
Italy	2.4	2.4	1.7	1.4	1.3	1.4
Latvia[2]	..	..	..	..	1.2	1.4
Lithuania	..	2.4	2.0	2.0	1.4	1.5
Luxembourg	2.3	2.0	1.5	1.6	1.8	1.6
Malta	..	..	2.0	2.0	1.7	1.4
Netherlands	3.1	2.6	1.6	1.6	1.7	1.8
Norway	2.9	2.5	1.7	1.9	1.9	2.0
Poland	3.0	2.2	2.3	2.0	1.4	1.4
Portugal	3.1	2.8	2.2	1.6	1.6	1.4
Romania	..	..	2.4	1.8	1.3	1.4
Slovak Republic	3.1	2.4	2.3	2.1	1.3	1.3
Slovenia	2.2	2.2	2.1	1.5	1.3	1.5
Spain	2.9	2.9	2.2	1.4	1.2	1.5
Sweden	2.2	1.9	1.7	2.1	1.6	1.9
Switzerland	2.4	2.1	1.6	1.6	1.5	1.5
Turkey	6.4	5.0	4.6	3.1	2.3	2.1
United Kingdom	2.7	2.4	1.9	1.8	1.6	2.0
EU	..	..	**2.0**	**1.8**	**1.5**	**1.6**

1. Data for Cyprus in 1980 refers to 1982.
2. Data for Latvia in 2000 refers to 2002.
Source: OECD Health Data 2010 and Eurostat Statistics Database.

StatLink http://dx.doi.org/10.1787/888932337718

Table A.5. **GDP per capita in 2008 and average annual growth rates, 1970 to 2008**

	GDP per capita in EUR at PPPs	Average annual growth rate (in real terms)			
	2008	1970-80	1980-90	1990-2000	2000-08
Austria	32 502	3.5	2.0	2.1	1.6
Belgium	30 834	3.2	1.9	1.9	1.5
Bulgaria	10 819	..	..	..	8.7
Cyprus	24 894	..	..	..	4.2
Czech Republic	21 482	..	..	0.3	4.3
Denmark	31 605	1.8	2.0	2.2	1.0
Estonia	17 713	..	..	..	6.9
Finland	30 768	3.4	2.6	1.7	2.6
France	28 435	3.0	1.9	1.6	0.9
Germany	30 411	2.7	2.1	0.3	1.2
Greece	24 841	3.6	0.2	1.6	3.6
Hungary	16 938	..	..	..	3.6
Iceland	31 747	5.3	1.6	1.5	2.5
Ireland	37 228	3.3	3.3	6.3	2.9
Italy	27 212	3.3	2.4	1.5	0.4
Latvia	15 037	..	..	..	9.4
Lithuania	16 285	..	..	..	9.5
Luxembourg	53 309	..	..	..	0.9
Malta	19 869	..	..	..	1.8
Netherlands	35 347	2.3	1.7	2.5	1.6
Norway	50 285	4.1	2.1	3.1	1.5
Poland	14 841	..	..	3.7	4.2
Portugal	19 986	3.5	3.0	2.6	0.5
Romania	12 559	..	..	..	11.7
Slovak Republic	19 045	..	..	..	6.2
Slovenia	23 992	..	..	..	4.1
Spain	27 775	2.5	2.6	2.4	1.9
Sweden	31 705	1.6	1.9	1.6	1.9
Switzerland	37 014	1.0	1.6	0.4	1.1
Turkey	11 388	..	..	1.7	3.0
United Kingdom	31 005	1.8	2.6	2.2	2.0
EU	**25 424**	**2.8**	**2.2**	**2.1**	**3.6**

Source: OECD Health Data 2010; Eurostat Statistics Database; WHO.

StatLink ᴍᴷᴸ http://dx.doi.org/10.1787/888932337737

ORGANISATION FOR ECONOMIC CO-OPERATION AND DEVELOPMENT

The OECD is a unique forum where governments work together to address the economic, social and environmental challenges of globalisation. The OECD is also at the forefront of efforts to understand and to help governments respond to new developments and concerns, such as corporate governance, the information economy and the challenges of an ageing population. The Organisation provides a setting where governments can compare policy experiences, seek answers to common problems, identify good practice and work to co-ordinate domestic and international policies.

The OECD member countries are: Australia, Austria, Belgium, Canada, Chile, the Czech Republic, Denmark, Finland, France, Germany, Greece, Hungary, Iceland, Ireland, Israel, Italy, Japan, Korea, Luxembourg, Mexico, the Netherlands, New Zealand, Norway, Poland, Portugal, the Slovak Republic, Slovenia, Spain, Sweden, Switzerland, Turkey, the United Kingdom and the United States. The European Commission takes part in the work of the OECD.

OECD Publishing disseminates widely the results of the Organisation's statistics gathering and research on economic, social and environmental issues, as well as the conventions, guidelines and standards agreed by its members.

OECD PUBLISHING, 2, rue André-Pascal, 75775 PARIS CEDEX 16
(81 2010 16 1 P) ISBN 978-92-64-09030-9 – No. 57505 2010